DR. VIGILANTE II

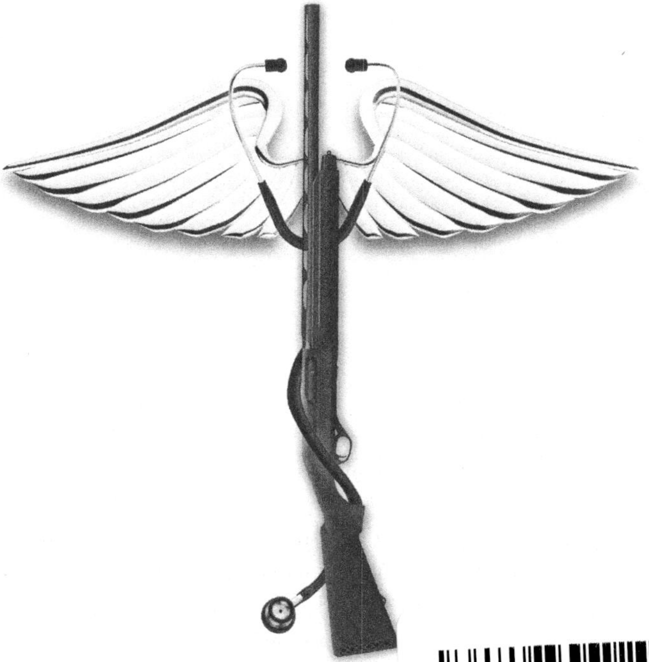

A Novel By

Alberto Hazan, MD

Cover design by Margo Murphy

ISBN: 978-0-9897909-8-7

When all the knots that strangle the heart are loosened,
the mortal becomes immortal.

—The Katha Upanishad

PART 1

Human Trafficking Statistics:

- *Human trafficking is the third largest criminal industry in the world, outranked only by arms and drug dealing.*[1] *It is known for the severe forms of violence it entails—such as incarceration, torture, rape, and sexual enslavement.*[2]
- *There are thirty million people in modern-day slavery across the world.*[3]
- *More than one million children are trafficked every year.*[4]
- *Up to ninety-five percent of victims experience physical and/or sexual violence during trafficking.*[5]
- *For every eight hundred people trafficked, only one person will be convicted.*[6]

---

1 *The Future Group, "Human Trafficking: A Human Security Crisis of Global Proportions."*

2 *United Nations Regional Information Centre, "Organs for Sale."*

3 *Fisher, Max. "This Map Shows Where The World's 30 Million Slaves Live." The Washington Post, October 17, 2013.*

4 *UNICEF, "Child Trafficking."*

5 *U.S. Department of Homeland Security, "Human Trafficking Awareness."*

6 *United Nations Global Initiative to Fight Human Trafficking, "Human Trafficking: The Facts."*

CHAPTER 1

Sound travels well in the humid air of the Guatemalan rainforest.

The hunter with the bow and arrow could have followed the two men ahead of him blindfolded. The tour guide's voice had grown loud and irritated in response to the constant whining of the clumsy American.

"You said a few more miles, Ernesto—wasn't that ten miles ago?"

"That was ten minutes ago, Señor."

"Ten minutes was two hours ago!"

"Not so loud, Señor Mel."

"Why not? There's nothing but trees around here."

"That may be," the guide said, lowering his voice to a rasp that the lean archer fifty feet away could still clearly hear. "But there are *traficantes* in this jungle. Traffickers. Drug and human. They find us, they may stuff us in sacks."

Mel Weiss stopped walking and fished out a sopping handkerchief. He wiped his forehead, which glistened anyway. "If the sack had air-conditioning, I wouldn't mind." His shirt was soaked in sweat and he was panting. He checked his TAG Heuer. "Six hours since we left Selaute, Ernesto. And every ten minutes you say, 'Just a few more miles.'" He plopped down and leaned back against a tree.

"Señor, slowly get away from that tree. Do not make any sudden movements."

"Just give me a second. I'm wiped out."

"I hear a rattle above you. "

Mel looked above him. "I hear leaves and branches."

"No, Señor. Poisonous snake sliding down. Bites your skin, you shake to death."

With a sudden nimbleness, Mel scooted behind Ernesto and looked back. A large ropey shadow writhed and dangled from the limb five feet above his resting place.

"Shake to death?" Mel chanted in a daze, then went on like the doctor he was, as if reciting symptoms. "You mean a seizure. Studied that on the flight. Rainforest snake venom. Highly neurotoxic. Half a milliliter in the blood, game over. Intractable seizures. Coagulation profile off the charts, leading to disseminated intravascular coagulopathy. Internal bleeding." He sounded disinterested, but then the full meaning of his words took effect. He scanned all the low tree limbs around him.

The surrounding jungle was thick with trees, but no more dangling snakes. "What about water snakes, Ernesto?" Mel looked around at the mossy terrain.

"Be calm now, Señor," Ernesto assured, cocking his head to the side and sniffing the air. "Nothing more nearby to worry us. I hear and smell no danger now."

"How can you tell for sure?"

"I grew up in this jungle, Señor Mel. I feed my family from here. I lead tours. I know every sound like you know with … your what-do-you-call-it?" He mimed listening to Mel's heart with an earpiece.

"Stethoscope?"

"Yes. Stethoscope. That's my jungle ear. Must move now. Night is coming soon. We cannot sleep here. Many dangerous creatures besides snakes."

"Like what?" Mel squeaked.

"Like all sorts of animals," Ernesto said. "But the *traficantes*. They are the most dangerous of all. Many of them around here now. Come—quiet and quickly."

Swigging from his water bottle, Mel walked right into a thorny bush.

"Ouch! Goddamn!" he yelled.

Ernesto clamped his hand over Mel's mouth, stifling his moans. "Shh, don't move."

"What are you doing?" Mel grunted.

"Shh!" Ernesto insisted.

Mel quieted. Ernesto took his hand away. They stood quietly for a moment, listening.

Late afternoon jungle sounds: the chirping of grasshoppers and beetles, the low buzz of dragonflies, the squabbling of toads, the swishing of giant leaves, the creaking of gently bending trunks, the splashing of unusually large bugs jumping in the watery moss—then a furious flapping overhead. A flock of dark-blue great curassow taking off from a high perch.

"They sound pissed," Mel said.

"Home invasion," Ernesto explained. "Wouldn't you be?" He resumed his brisk pace, and Mel waddled to catch up, picking thorns from his pants.

"Talk low, now, Señor. You say where to take you, but not why."

Mel gulped more water, then poured some over his sweaty head and rubbed his face with his chubby hands. "I came here for help."

"*Si?*"

"That's right, Ernesto. A matter of life and death."

Ernesto cut Mel a look of sudden concern. "Someone you know, Señor?"

"Oh yeah," Mel said, grateful for Ernesto's intuition. "Someone back home. She's in bad shape. In a coma the last two weeks."

"What is wrong with this señorita?"

"Nobody knows," Mel said, his voice barely above a whisper. "She's in critical condition. The doctors at St. Jude's—the hospital where I work—they've done all sorts of tests, but nobody has a clue. No viable diagnosis. I'm here to find the only person I know who can figure out what's wrong with her and maybe save her before it's too late."

"In Guatemala?" Ernesto asked, incredulously. "Here, in the jungle?"

"I know," Mel said. "Hard to believe, but true. There's a doctor from New York who moved here two months ago. He may be certifiably insane, but he's the best doctor I've ever known. I was told he lives in that village I showed you on the map ..."

"Shh." Ernesto raised his hand.

"What's wrong?" Mel looked up at the trees. "Another snake?"

Ernesto didn't say anything. He squinted upward, then toward the tree the archer had slipped behind.

The archer made no move.

After a moment, Ernesto's voice broke the silence. "More birds, I think. Come on. Just a few more miles."

"I've heard that before," Mel grumbled, plodding on.

A half hour later, Ernesto pointed excitedly. "That river I know! Water for the village. Just past those Ceiba trees."

Mel wiped his face with his shirt hem. He looked at the flying shadows above the trees and gave a grim smile. "Those are big birds. Pretty yellow heads."

"King Vultures," Ernesto said. "I'm not liking this."

"I'm not a fan of vultures," Mel said. "They're the last birds I want on my welcoming committee."

As they trekked through the Ceiba grove, a dank aroma grew stronger. They emerged from the trees and stopped dead. They stared at the remains of the village, burnt to the ground. Dozens of thatched wooden houses had been destroyed, the blackened wood posts standing alone in piles of mud wall fragments. Heaps of charred clothing were scattered throughout the former village. There was nothing but rubble and ashes and the smell of death.

"I … don't … understand," Ernesto fumbled. "The village … It was here six months ago. I took a tour group. They stayed here overnight. Hiked the next day to Kundal, the Mayan ruins. It's the main stop for tourists who come to Selaute. It's what they do. This … is … tragic."

"What the hell happened here?" Mel struggled to catch his breath. "How could … but this means …" With a wheeze he found his voice. "My sources told me Robert was here. The Selaute people said they saw him enter the jungle two months ago. They recognized his picture. White man walking, hiking here, they said. Right around New Year's. Saw him go in the jungle." Mel squatted and buried his head in his hands. "He didn't die in the jungle, did he? Or get burned to death here? What are we going to do?"

"I'm so sorry, Señor. This is all so confusing. Let me think. I didn't hear of any fires. Maybe the *traficantes* burned the village down. We have to go back to Selaute first thing tomorrow morning. We cannot go back now. We will set up camp here, sleep, wake tomorrow and begin to return."

The archer had joined up with two others. All three shared a smile when they heard the American tourist exhale like a snorting pig. The archer raised his bow and drew back the string in one graceful motion. His eyes grew merry as he sighted the tourist raising his fancy water bottle.

With a fearsome snap and gusty whoosh, the arrow shot off on a twenty-yard hardline journey.

CHAPTER 2

As Mel brought the water bottle up to his lips, a long black arrow shot through it, propelling it violently from his hands and pinning it to a tree a few feet away. Water trickled to the ground.

"*Que hacen aquí, pendejos?*" boomed a rough Spanish voice.

With a rustle of leaves, a young muscular man in cargo pants emerged, smeared with black paint patterns on his face and shirtless torso. He had an arrow aimed right between Mel's jumping eyes.

Ernesto trembled, his face ashen.

A second man appeared, this one shorter, skinnier, barely twenty years old. The kid had a sunken midchest—a pectus excavatum—and held a spear. He walked right up to Mel and pointed its metal blade at his face.

"*Que haces aquí?*"

Mel could only stammer. "I … um … don't speak Español."

Ernesto rasped. "He asked—"

"*Callate pendejo,*" the kid barked, whopping Ernesto's cheek with the flat of the blade, then quickly re-aiming the spear at Mel. "What's your name, gringo?" he asked with a confident American accent, bringing the spear-point within a millimeter of Mel's eye.

"Please, don't hurt me," Mel pleaded. "I'm just a tourist. I mean no harm."

"I asked you a question."

"My name is Mel Weiss. I'm a doctor. Emergency physician. From New York."

"New York?" the leader repeated. "Now in Guatemala? City man sweating like a roasting boar now in the jungle? You're not a tourist. One lie, one cut." With a deft flick, he drew a small red line of blood on Mel's jowl. "What are you really doing here? You lie again, I'll cut you deeper."

Mel didn't make a noise. He placed the back of his hand against the cut to stanch the flow of blood. "All truth," he said. "No problem. I'm looking for a man—an American doctor I know. He can help my wife. She's sick in New York. In a coma. She's been like that for the past two weeks. In the intensive care unit. No one knows what's wrong with her. This doctor I know, who lives here, I worked with him. He's very smart. Brilliant diagnostician—he can help, I think. He's my only hope. That's why I came here, to the jungle. Maybe you know him. An American doctor?"

"*Es verdad,*" Ernesto confirmed. "*El doctor Weiss busca su colega.*"

The kid gave a sharp nod to his cohort, who turned his drawn bow on Ernesto, digging the arrow tip into the fleshy part of his neck, but not breaking the skin. "Do not use your throat again for talk," the cohort said in his deep, piercing voice. "Gringo slave! Giving white men our jungle for their phone pictures. Click, click!"

"My friend here doesn't like tourists, or the U.S. much," the kid said to Mel. "And you say 'American' doctor, like you own America. But we are American, not just you."

"You're right," Mel sputtered. "Absolutely. A U.S. doctor. I apologize."

"What is the name of this doctor?"

"Robert McKenzie."

A fleeting look of recognition lit the young archer's face.

"You know him?" Mel cried.

The boy shook his head.

"Please," Mel begged. "You know him. I saw it on your face. Please! My wife needs help. She's dying. Where is he? Where's Robert?"

The tears welling in Mel's eyes drowned his fear. He was now a man simply doing all he could to help someone he desperately loved, and the boy could see that. His expression remained stoic for a while, but then the boy broke into a smile. He started chuckling. His cohort added his deep rumbling laughter.

Mel's eyes widened and lit up, clearly taking the change in mood as a good sign. "So," Mel started, hesitantly, "you know where he is. Can you take me to Robert?"

"I don't think you want me to do that, fat man."

"No, it's okay," Mel said, unfazed by the insult. "He'll want to see me, I promise. We're good friends. He'll be happy to see me."

"No, I promise you he wouldn't say that." The kid's grin turned into a sneer.

"Well, I don't know if he'd be happy to see me. He might be surprised at first. I guess he might be angry with me. I had to fire him a couple of months ago. But I think he's forgiven me. And he knows my wife, so I'm sure he's going to want to help. We've had dinners together, been to parties. Please! She's dying. I wouldn't be here otherwise."

The boy had no smile now. He just stared at Mel, saying nothing.

"If you won't lead me to him, at least tell me where he is," Mel pressed on.

"He's underground."

Mel's jaw fell. The kid looked back at him steadily, and then looked slowly around at the long shadows the setting sun cast from the ruins of the village.

"By underground," Mel said. "You mean ...?"

"I mean dead. We killed him last week." The boy lowered the spear and moved closer to Mel's face. "We hunted him like a boar, caught him in a net, tied his hands and feet together, threw a rope over that tree where your water bottle is pinned, then pulled him up by his limbs until he cried himself to death. Which is what we're now going to do to you."

"What? No! How could you do that to Robert?" Mel yelled, lifting his hands before him, his voice quivering. "Please. There's no need to ... um ... this is just, all so ... horrible. We're no threat. I just came here to find my friend."

"Easy to say, gringo. But you could be lying. What are so many foreign doctors doing in our jungle? Why are you really here? Are you working with the *traficantes*? Are you a soldier?"

"Me? A soldier? Look at me, for Christ's sake. I'm sixty-two, a hundred pounds overweight, blind without these Coke-bottle glasses. I nearly had a thrombotic stroke hiking these last six miles."

"Maybe you are not a soldier," the kid said, "but maybe a soldier's doctor. Our spies report extra doctors now in the enemy camp. This is new. And it can't be good. We can't take a chance with either of you. But it's not all bad. You'll meet your precious Robert very soon now in the underground." He nodded to his cohort. "*Vamos*, Miguel. Hog-tie these fools."

"No!" Ernesto cried. "*Por favor. Yo soy inocente.*"

Mel began crying and sank to the ground in a pool of his own urine.

From the woods behind them a voice bellowed in perfect Spanish. "*Ya es suficiente!*"

The kid and his cohort stepped back five paces, lowered their weapons and smiled.

A figure emerged from the foliage—the lean archer himself. His bow's elegant waxed curvature caught golden glints from the setting sun. His quiver was full of long arrows as dark as the gathering shadows. He was in full camouflage, wearing a hoodie and high-tech glasses.

He walked as quietly as a stalking panther up to Mel and yanked him upright. He then lowered the hoodie and took off his glasses.

"Welcome to the jungle, old friend," Robert said with a smile. "Did you miss me?"

CHAPTER 3

"Goddamn it, Robert!" Mel yelled. "How could you? That's low, even for you. Just … plain … cruel."

"Now you know how I felt when you fired me," Robert said evenly. He had never seen his former boss so angry. Mel Weiss, esteemed director of St. Jude Hospital's Emergency Department, was known for his aplomb and rationality in that high-stress environment. But now his face was hot-sauce red, and spittle bubbled on his lips. His pants were soaked with urine and he was barely choking down a primal growl.

Robert held his gaze, letting Mel see in his eyes the pain his firing had caused. He was upset at being ripped from patients who would die without his expertise, at being catapulted from New York City. He missed his secret double life treating patients in the ER during the day and decimating the city's psychotic criminal population at night.

He saw the old Mel slowly returning, probably as Mel read these feelings in Robert. The redness faded from his quivering jowls. Mel wiped his mouth, sighed loudly and hung his head. "I'm sorry, Robert, for the damage I caused you. Truly. I really am." He looked up, and Robert felt a pang when he saw tears mix with the drops of sweat on Mel's face. "But it's Francine. She might be dying. She's been in a coma for the past thirteen days. No one knows why."

"I overheard, Mel. I'm sorry." Robert placed a hand on Mel's shoulder. "Is that really why you came here?"

Mel stared at Robert. "You're my last hope."

Robert nodded. "We've been down this road before, remember? I diagnosed Francine when nobody else could. We'll get on it. I promise."

Mel gave a hesitant smile.

"By the way, despite your lack of physical endurance, you actually look a bit healthier. You've lost some weight."

"I have. Worrying about Francine. Not hungry all the time like before."

"Yeah, stress will do that. It also accounts for your orbits looking so sunken," Robert said. "And look at you. Hirsutism hit you at the sixth decade of life."

Mel's eyes brightened, catching on to the familiarity. "Oh yeah," he said, fingering his scraggly beard. "Shaving just got to seem like too much work. But look who's talking. That beard can use a serious trim."

"I guess." Robert wrinkled his nose. "When's the last time you washed?"

Mel shrugged. "I should've taken a nice long hot shower at the InterContinental in Guatemala City, but I was in a hurry to find you. How was I to know it'd be my last shot at indoor plumbing for two days? I guess I thought there'd be decent accommodations in Selaute or the surrounding villages. Ha! Critters in the water and toilet pits. Isn't this supposed to be a touristy spot? I sure didn't expect to find your new digs in a real jungle."

"Not many tourists around here any more. The Kundal ruins are closed for restoration and the disgusting violence in this area is getting even worse." Robert yanked his arrow out of the tree, ripped off the water bottle and tossed it to Mel. "Souvenir!"

Mel caught it, looked at it, then dropped it on the ground. "No thanks."

Ernesto pounced on the bottle and quickly stuffed it in his backpack. "You shouldn't litter in our home."

"You're absolutely right," Mel said. "I'm sorry."

"Thanks, Ernesto," Robert said. "By the way, I'm sorry for involving you in all this."

"*No hay problema*, Doctor Robert," Ernesto said with a big smile. "I know I take risks introducing gringos like yourself to our jungle."

"Ouch," Robert said with a laugh. He smoothed the arrow's feathers and slid it back in his quiver.

"And what's with this bow and arrow crap, Robert?" Mel asked. "Since when are you the hunting type?"

"There's a lot you don't know about me."

"Well, I can guess. You're worried about the bad guys around here, right? So get a gun. Bow and arrow? Seriously, it's the twenty-first century. Why the rudimentary weapons?"

"To prevent pollution. Noise and land pollution. You don't want to scare animals, and you especially don't want to give our location to all the narco-terrorists and traffickers around here."

"Okay. Got it. And it's easier, I guess, to make spears and bows in the jungle than guns."

"Don't underestimate what you can get from this jungle, Mel. In fact, we've built a huge arsenal of weapons we confiscated from all the *traficantes* we've ambushed. Enough to stock a small army."

"I didn't realize how many of those bastards there are around here." Mel looked around nervously. "Is that why your Neanderthal friend there attacked us? He thought we were drug dealers?"

Immediately, the boy with the pectus excavatum marched up to Mel and got in his face. "Maybe you're throwing the word 'Neanderthal' around a little too easily, Señor."

"Easy, Armando," Robert said. "Give the dumb gringo a little breathing space. Dr. Weiss doesn't realize how well you and the other villagers understand English. And Spanish. And K'iche'. How many languages do you speak, Mel?"

"God, I'm sorry. I was way out of line there, Armando."

"All right," Robert said. "Let's get a move on." He took Mel's heavy bag from him and slung it around his shoulder. "It's kind of a trek to our village and it's getting dark. You ready?"

Mel nodded, a sunken look appearing again on his face.

"It's okay," Robert said. "I know how strange this all must be for you. Let's walk and catch up."

CHAPTER 4

Robert led Mel and Ernesto out of the ghost village. Armando and Miguel melted into the forest behind them, a pair of invisible bodyguards hidden by the surrounding foliage.

For five minutes, Mel trudged along in silence behind Robert on an unmarked trail, then called out, "Slow down, Robert. Let me catch my breath for a moment." He stopped, put his hands on his knees and panted a bit.

Robert stopped without turning around. He studied his surroundings. When he was sure there was no imminent danger, he walked back and squatted by Mel.

"You okay, old man?"

"Yeah," Mel said, after a bit. "You know, you've probably lost more weight than I have."

Robert forced a smile. Mel had no idea what he'd been through, or what the villagers in this jungle had suffered.

The torture, the abuse, the kidnappings, the rapes.

"It's tough staying alive here, Mel—sometimes even wanting to stay alive."

Mel held his gaze for a long beat, then nodded. "Seems that way. Maybe it's time to come back home. I don't like to see you looking so beaten down."

"I'm not beaten, Mel. Count on that."

"I hope not."

"I came here to get away from the chaos of the city," Robert said. "I needed a few months to recharge. Instead, I've done nothing but help protect these jungles against the *traficantes*."

"Funny how the ones who take care of others aren't always able to take care of themselves." He grabbed a handful of belly fat. "Well, thanks for the breather. Let's get going."

They started walking again, this time side by side. "It's good to see you, Mel," Robert said. "I missed your wide-load Big Apple charm."

"Yeah, right," Mel said, trying to keep pace.

"I did." Robert pulled out his machete and cut three thick vines with one swipe. "So tell me about Francine."

"She's real sick, Robert. I wouldn't be disturbing you otherwise."

"I get that," Robert said. "It's not endocarditis again, is it?"

"No, that's the first thing we ruled out. We did a trans-esophageal echocardiogram. Heart valves were perfect. Everything was. Her ejection fraction. Her blood cultures. Cardiac enzymes, BNP, D-dimer, ESR, CRP—all normal. CAT scans, MRIs, PET scans—normal. Toxicology screen—negative. On paper, my wife is in perfect health. She just doesn't seem to be able to open her goddamn eyes any more. Ever since I found her two weeks ago."

"Found her how?"

"When I came home from work one night, I found her lying on the floor by the bed, unresponsive. Shook her, yelled at her. Sternal rub—couldn't wake her up. She was still breathing fine and had a bounding pulse, but she just wouldn't respond. Finally I called 911, then a full siren run to St. Jude's. Worst ride of my life! Gave me too good an idea of what she'd look like dead. It was terrible, Robert." Mel choked back tears. "We pulled into the ambulance bay and I get this crushing feeling—no Robert in the ER anymore. I had eighty-sixed Francine's only hope. You not being there made me feel like I'd dug my own wife's grave."

"Let me guess," Robert said, "Dr. Valentine saw her and ordered the full panel."

There was a beat of silence as Mel clamped his mouth shut and fought back tears, staring at a slice of horizon peeking through the thickly tangled jungle. "Valentine's a robot! You could've diagnosed her in half an hour with a tenth of the workup."

Robert put his arm around his former boss for a few paces. "It's okay, Mel."

"I have so many regrets."

"You shouldn't regret firing me. You had to. You really did. And remember, I gave you my resignation letter anyway."

"Yeah, maybe. But I don't care what you say—I'm guilty of not standing up for you. I should never have listened to the rest of the staff. Hacks! I was responsible for firing St. Jude's best diagnostician, and now karma is biting my big fat ass."

"All in the past, Mel. Nothing can change that."

"Something can sure as hell change the future. We can, damn it! Even before those blubbering residents finished all their stabs in the dark, I knew I'd have to find you somehow and drag you back to St. Jude's. Robert, I want you to take your old job back. Let me make amends for my past mistakes."

Robert smiled. He wasn't sure if Mel's outburst came from regret or desperation. But one thing was true: Mel meant every word he said.

The other truth was that Robert really did deserve to be fired. His vigilantism had made him reckless. He'd left an emergency room full of critical patients in his bloodthirst to avenge those kids tortured and killed by the neo-Nazis. He could've waited a few hours and still decimated those psychopaths. Despite his best intentions, Robert needed expulsion from the whole scene, a forced vacation from the grueling life he'd carved for himself in New York, slaving over patients in the chaos of the ER by day and hunting down child molesters, rapists, and wife-beaters by night.

"How'd you find me, Mel? Only a couple people knew my whereabouts."

"And I talked to them both," Mel said. "Nurse Rivera told me you were in Guatemala, but it was the social worker, Reede, who gave me the details. She told me to go to Selaute and ask for Roberto. Very helpful girl, that Reede. She's got a beautiful soul."

Robert nodded calmly while a volcano awoke in his chest. He burned and flooded with the sudden admission of a fact he'd been resisting ever since he emigrated: Sharon Reede, the ER social worker at St. Jude's, was the best thing that'd ever happened to him. She had found her way inside his cocoon—somehow cracked and tunneled through his defensive barrier, the armor he kept around his heart to keep anyone from hurting it further, including himself. Lockboxing his chest had allowed him to focus on avenging those in need without emotional distraction.

But Sharon found the key to that lockbox.

She was the key.

She'd been able to get close because she genuinely cared about him. Her uncanny intelligence had led her to uncover his secret identity as the Manhattan Vigilante. She'd figured out that he lived a double life—emergency physician by day, vigilante by night.

The admiration in Mel's voice when he spoke of her lit a fire under Robert that he thought he'd smothered.

But right now he couldn't let it burn. He had some terrifying unfinished business left in Guatemala. One moment of inattention could have unspeakable results for him and his new community.

He rubbed his face vigorously, trying to smooth it from all traces of worry and yearning. Even as he turned a stoic look toward Mel, fantasies of returning with him to New York and surprising Sharon in her apartment reeled in his mind.

He made his voice as hard as he wanted his resolve to be.

"Mel, I need the whole picture of you finding Francine if you want me to help. Walk me through it. Let me feel it out, see what triggers an alarm. It's how I do this stuff. Tell me what led up to you getting home and the details of her lying on the floor."

Mel stared at the distance. A pack of howler monkeys made a heart-jolting ruckus above them, but neither Mel nor Robert bothered to look up.

"Actually," Mel began, "that day was a pretty big one for me in the ER. At a budget meeting, I had finally convinced the CEO that overcrowding was seriously screwing up his sacred bottom line. The clincher was this article I quoted from the *Annals of Emergency Medicine* about how increased boarding in the ER leads to more deaths, longer stays and, more important to the suits, higher costs. Soaring! You should have seen that little prick's eye sparkle at that. Saving money? Alert the media! It was beautiful. I finally got through to him. He was going to take my findings back to the money-grubbing administrators who design hospital policy. Huge win for me, the ER, and all our patients. I was feeling great. Couldn't wait to share the news with my wife and cheer her up. She'd been kind of distant lately."

"For how long?" Robert interjected quickly.

"Oh!" Mel looked startled. "A while."

"Be more specific."

"At least five or six months."

"Why had she been distant?"

"I think it's because she doesn't sleep well. Bad insomnia. Her medications aren't working lately. I wake up in the middle of the night to go to the bathroom and she's lying there, eyes wide open. She's tired a lot. I can't seem to get her to want to do anything fun lately."

"Why'd you think your budget news would cheer her up?"

"I bought a dozen roses, a box of Godiva, and her favorite Pinot Noir to help things along. But when I got home ..." He stopped suddenly, his voice quivering.

Robert homed in—they were working, no time for sentiment. "So you found her lying on the floor next to the bed? Like she had fallen off?"

"Yeah," Mel said, swiping quickly at his eyes. He knew the drill. "She was completely unresponsive. Breathing, though. Maintaining her airway fine. No respiratory distress. No cyanosis. At first I thought maybe a stroke, checked her pulse for A-Fib. Nope. Pulse regular. Looked around for empty pill bottles. None. Signs of trauma? Nothing. So I called the paramedics."

Mel couldn't keep in his sobs any longer, and Robert gave him a breather.

Something wasn't adding up, but Robert couldn't figure out what.

Mel was quiet again, blowing his nose onto the forest floor. He caught Robert's smile, and said, "What?"

"It's okay, Mel," Robert said. "Jungle hanky. We use them all the time."

Mel laughed in spite of his misery. "Biodegradable too, right?"

As Robert spied the grove of guava trees that meant his village was near, his mind whirled with images and scenes wrought by Mel's story. A vision in which he saw Mel drop the roses on the floor next to the sad but kind face of Francine, whom Robert had met a number of times. She was lying on the floor, unconscious.

No trauma. No pills. No disease.

A clicking chorus of giant insects rose like bats from a tangle of vines ahead of them and scattered Robert's thoughts into the humid air, leaving him with the sense of an idea he couldn't quite grasp.

What am I missing?

"I wish I could've called you, Robert," Mel said, "instead of that damn 911. Or e-mailed you—even texted you. But apparently social media is not your thing anymore. You've gone all anti-tech on me."

Robert's lips curled into a smile. "Don't take it personal, Mel. I haven't logged on or smartphoned or keyboarded since I came here. My computer and cell are sitting happy as frogs on a log in a bank deposit box in Guatemala City. These wilds are world enough for me. The twitters here are all natural. Closest to peace a maniac like me could ever hope for."

"You must miss something in New York. People there, conveniences, the challenging medical cases? Hell, even the whip-smart suits bouncing by with their briefcases and sultry glares?"

"There's something rotten in the U.S., and I don't see anything left there for me but spin doctors, ulterior motives, and broken promises."

"It's not all that bad."

Robert grimaced. He knew Mel was right. If he were being honest, Robert wanted to be back in New York City more than anything.

And for only one reason.

He wondered if there were any messages from Sharon waiting for him in his inbox. Maybe he should make a quick trip to the capital. At times she haunted him even more than the recent violence in the jungle.

Does she ever think about me? Is she seeing someone else?

But he'd left his computer in Guatemala City on purpose. He was afraid he'd weaken and reach out to her. Besides making him personally exposed, this might also make him vulnerable to the authorities. It might alert eavesdropping police still looking for him as a person of concern in the neo-Nazi warehouse incident.

And yet Robert had been away for a couple of months. By now Macy and Landers, the two detectives who had checked him out, were no doubt swamped by a new caseload. Besides, Landers was sympathetic. He'd given Robert the opportunity to escape, urging him to leave New York. Surely, he wouldn't dog him if he returned.

Especially if it was just for one night with Sharon.

"Seriously, Robert," Mel said, "don't you want your old job back? We need you back, that's for damn sure. And believe it or not, there are a few people other than your BFF Rivera who miss you."

"I'm not saying I won't consider going back," Robert said. "But if it's to help Francine get better, I can do it from here. I'm assuming you brought all the lab results and imaging studies?"

"I did," Mel exulted.

"The original scans, not the radiology reports."

Mel pointed to his backpack. “It’s all here, Robert. Thank you. Really.”

They emerged into the clearing of the village after slogging through several barriers of thick foliage that had completely hidden it from sight. The huts were close together. The small but teeming population consisted mostly of young women and children. There were a few men, some of whom were going about their business: chopping wood for the fire, plucking chickens, simmering broth. Kids played with a makeshift soccer ball made of twigs, dried moss, mud, and sap. A middle-aged man was instructing several teenagers on how to use a bow and arrow.

Robert swept his hand high, and Armando and Miguel materialized as if from the marshy ground. With a curt nod at Robert, they escorted Ernesto into the village, while Robert held Mel back.

“There are a few rules I have to lay down before you enter our community.” Robert watched the villagers greet the new arrivals. He paused and turned to Mel. “But before I do, tell me why you cheated on Francine.”

CHAPTER 5

"How did you know?" Mel asked, his face ashen.

"That's not pertinent," Robert said. "I want to know *why*. Francine's a special woman. A good wife, a great mother. Why did you do it?"

Mel turned from Robert and lowered his gaze. A burst of laughter rose from the group gathered around Armando, and Mel ran his hands through his sweaty hair. Behind him, the jungle was a maze of darkening greens and brown.

"What the hell, Robert?" Mel erupted. "That was unreal. How did you figure it out? I need to know."

Robert shrugged. "It was a guess, Mel, but pretty well founded. And it looks like you just confirmed it. When did it start? Six months ago?"

"Come on, Robert. I know it wasn't a guess. Just tell me."

"You mentioned earlier that Francine had started acting distant a few months ago. Probably you were the one being distant, projecting it on her. She has trouble sleeping and you randomly bring her flowers and Pinot Noir? There's a lot you're not telling me."

"That sounds like something the ER social worker would say."

"No doubt," Robert said, secretly liking the accusation but keeping a poker face. "I might've picked up a bit of her jargon along the way. But also—you coming here? Lording your way through the jungle to find me? Not something the Mel I knew would normally do. Guilt drove you to Guatemala."

"Not guilt as much as concern and love for my wife. You're the only one who can help."

"She's in a stable condition, Mel. Comatose yes, but only for two weeks. Not life-threatening yet. You need to start being honest with me. Just admit that you've been cheating on her and that guilt drove you to find me." Robert paused for a moment, but then plowed on. "It's the only explanation that makes sense. You're such a responsible administrator—for all your bellyaching, you love that ER. Especially now, since you're all excited about getting the CEO on your side for the budget. You've always hated missing work, especially in March with all its staff meetings, budget wrangling, new hires, Passover. I figured only terrible guilt could cattle-prod you out of there and drive your fat ass through snakes and quicksand to find me. I know how much your wife means to you, but you would've made arrangements. You would've been more patient with the workup and the consultants. At the very least, you wouldn't drop everything to trek across the hemisphere to find me. That's guilt. Bone-crushing, ball-shrinking, heart-wrenching guilt."

Mel stayed quiet. His face turned a sickly yellow.

"Look, Mel, I'm not going to give you a lecture about the virtues of being faithful, or the hell bites of infidelity. I'm sure you know plenty more about that than I do. I'm just here to help you figure out what happened to your wife. Period. You can deal with the aftereffects when she gets better. Okay?"

Mel nodded solemnly. "I quit the affair that night. The roses and wine were guilt offerings, really. I left the hospital feeling all wired about the CEO meeting and went straight to my mistress, a former secretary."

"Who's that?"

Mel remained silent.

"For crying out loud, don't tell me it was Allison?"

Mel just winced.

Robert rolled his eyes, but he didn't say anything further. He could sense Mel's growing disgust at the cesspool he'd been splashing around in. Allison was a cleavage-proud money-grubber. Francine was a modest, shapely, loving woman.

"All right, Mel. Go on."

"Yeah. So I knock on Allison's door, feeling all bright and revved, like everything's coming together, you know. She lets me in and I see how messy her house is, as usual. Then she starts going on and on about how much she hates her colleagues and her job and her family. Something awoke in me that had been hibernating. I came out of my own coma, I guess, and realized how little I wanted to be there, let alone to have sex with that woman. I told her it was over and she threw a glass vase at me. Luckily she missed. Then I left. Bought some roses and wine and hightailed it home. The night before I'd told Francine I was going to a medical conference in New Orleans, when I was really planning a trip to Las Vegas with Allison. On my way home, I pictured how happy Francine would be to hear that I'd canceled the trip. I could feel all my love for her rising up again. I was going to spoil her. I was going to be a different person. I was going to be the real Mel—Francine's Mel." At this point, his voice choked, and he slammed the side of his fist against the tree they were under.

"Okay. I get it. But for now, you've got to focus," Robert said. "I need more details about how you found her. I'm not quite seeing what you saw when you got home. How was she lying on the floor? Was there anything out of place in the room?"

"She had knocked over the bedside table" Mel straightened up. "My guess is she grabbed onto it when she felt herself falling and pulled it over. No signs of head trauma, though."

"Give me more details. I have to walk that room in your shoes."

"Um, well, I found our honeymoon picture. It had fallen behind the table. I hadn't even noticed it was gone until a month or so ago. The glass in the frame was cracked—from falling, I guess. And ..." Mel choked up again.

"And what?"

"Nothing. It's just a little irony, that's all. Her wedding ring was under the bed near the picture."

"Her ring? Had it rolled off her finger?"

"No," Mel said. "She had sprained her knuckle a while back. Her ring-finger knuckle. In the gym while doing weights. Her finger was swollen and sore so she'd taken the ring off and placed it on the bedside table."

Robert grew quiet as he registered the additional information. There was something not adding up.

Too many missing pieces.

"Okay," Robert said. "I got enough background. Let's see the goods."

"I brought all the lab and imaging stuff." Mel opened his bag and showed Robert a jumble of papers inside. "EKG, EEG, MRI, CT, CBC, CMP, U/A, ESR, CRP, Utox."

"Great. Don't worry, Mel, I'll figure it out. Like I said, we've been down this road before."

Mel's eyes filled with tears. "Thank you, Robert. You helped Francine so much in the past, diagnosing her subacute bacterial endocarditis when nobody else could—and now you're doing it again. It was poor judgment to fire you."

"You can rehire me once I figure out what's wrong with her."

"I'd do that and more. I'm going to tell the board to give a raise to that social worker, Reede, too. She's been incredible."

Robert surged with adrenaline hearing Sharon's name, and at that moment he made up his mind. As soon as he finished his business in Guatemala, he'd return to New York and surprise Sharon when she least expected it. Then he'd stay with her as long as she wanted.

"She's really supportive," Mel went on. "She's got this killer schedule, but every night she's in the ICU, sitting by Francine's side. And she's so nice to me, so comforting."

"Yes, she is."

"When I expressed to her how much I wished you were around to help Francine, she told me where you were. I think I surprised her by immediately pulling out my cellphone and buying a plane ticket."

"Did she ask you to give me any messages? A note or something?"

"No," he said. "Should she have?"

"No. Just wondering."

"Uh-huh." Mel looked at Robert speculatively.

An uncomfortable silence settled between them.

"Okay, Mel." Robert steered the conversation back to the task at hand. "Let me give you a quick tour of the village. Then we can get you something to eat, and I'll start looking at these charts. You must be starving after your long trek.

And listen, I know it won't come natural, but try to act humble. People here are leery of foreigners."

"Humble? It's my natural state. The humblest guy the world has ever known!"

"Proud and humble."

"I can handle that," Mel said, saluting facetiously.

Robert shook his head and led Mel to the large fire in the middle of the village, tended by a gray-haired man in his late sixties built like a professional wrestler. As they walked, all the villagers seemed to pause and watch their progress. Only the elder feeding the large fire didn't seem to notice them. His fierce eyes stayed fixed on the dancing flames.

Robert and Mel stopped two yards behind the man, who didn't turn.

"Mel," Robert said in a louder than usual voice. "Let me introduce you to Guillermo. The medicine man."

CHAPTER 6

"You know our policy about bringing strangers to the village, don't you Roberto?" the man said without taking his eyes off the fire.

"This guy is no stranger, Guillermo. He's a friend. My former boss."

Guillermo slowly turned and looked Mel up and down without a trace of friendliness. "Another doctor?"

"That's right." Robert patted Mel on the back.

"Dr. Weiss." Mel offered a hand. "Pleasure to meet you, Guillermo. I guess you head your medicine department, just like I do back home."

Guillermo stared at the hand. "Do you really expect me to shake your hand? A hand you haven't washed for at least two days? A hand that's probably touched all kinds of filthy things—bacteria-infected things—like your unwashed genitals?" He looked at Robert. "Your country's idea of what is civilized rarely passes the gates of reason. You continue to grind unwashed palms together whenever you meet, despite Semmelweis's research over a century ago. I can read your thoughts, Dr. Weiss. You may think me a primitive witch doctor, but at least I know hygiene."

Mel dropped his gaze and put his hands in his pockets, looking awkward and uncomfortable.

Robert hadn't expected a friendly encounter, just an entertaining one. Guillermo hated to meet new people, and lately he'd been less trusting in general. His medical and fighting skills, though, were still first rate.

"Wipe that smile off your face, Roberto! You, Armando and Miguel were supposed to bring back dinner an hour ago. Instead, you bring back this overweight American and his tour guide. Two more mouths to feed and no food?"

Robert's smile straightened. "Don't worry, Guillermo. I'll be back in fifteen minutes with the village's meals."

"You better. I just made the fire and our food better be here before it goes out."

Robert's eyes danced like the flames. He loved a challenge, especially from Guillermo.

"Armando!" Robert called.

Twenty yards away, Armando stroked some bare-breasted beauty's hair. He whirled around expectantly.

"Let's go hunt that lovely lady some dinner," Robert said.

The young woman clapped and flashed a brilliant smile. Armando gave her a quick kiss on the cheek and trotted over.

Mel hissed to Robert. "You're not leaving me alone with this guy. I'm coming with you."

"Suit yourself. But keep up. Guillermo's word is law here. We're on the clock."

Robert led Mel and Armando away from the fire pit—the center of the circling village—to the largest hut on the rim, guarded by a muscular young man who bumped fists with each of them as they passed. Mel shook his sore hand with a scowl after the fist bump, but the scowl quickly turned to astonishment when he noticed the arsenal inside.

Hundreds of firearms, machine guns, assault rifles. All types of knives and spears. High-tech radios and accessories. Spy equipment, satellite phones.

"Holy shit," Mel sputtered. "What is all this?"

"Enough weapons to equip a small army," Robert said. "Which is what we need here. We got this arsenal from the drug dealers who infest these parts of the woods—narcotraficantes. We strip them of their weapons, take their boots, bloody them and leave them to make their way back to Guatemala City by foot. Most of them don't make it out of the jungle. If the jaguars don't get them, the snakes or skeeters do."

"Jesus, Robert, isn't that a bit harsh for some poor natives just moving some coke around ..."

"Who will shoot you if they see you first," Armando interjected. "Besides, they're not just trafficking drugs any more. They do people now. Young girls, especially."

"Sex trade?" Mel asked.

"These guys don't have souls," Robert explained. "They've expanded from drugs into kidnapping. Human trafficking in Central and South America has gone sky-high, especially in Guatemala and Mexico. These assholes go into poor villages, wherever they can, and grab people—especially young girls—and then sell them to the sex industry or God knows where else. It's a lucrative trade, and this area seems to be one of their happiest hunting grounds. Because they've closed off Kundal from tourists, there are fewer armed guards around. The jackals think they have carte blanche. We've managed to rescue a few victims and get some proper pay-back, but every week more of our neighbors are hit, men are killed, women are raped, and children are dragged kicking and screaming into slavery and prostitution."

As Mel digested all this with a look of horror on his face, Robert scrounged for what he needed. He was going boar hunting and wanted his pet bow, the one he'd brought here from the U.S.

His famed recurve bow.

Most hunters shot with a high-tech compound bow. Its complex series of fiber optic sights, stabilizers, and gadgets made for better accuracy. Robert preferred the old-fashioned recurve. Nothing but bow and string. It took more skill to aim by feel, but Robert had that skill and loved that feel. He thought it was disrespectful to the animal to use the compound for hunting. It was an unfair advantage.

Robert found the bow hidden where he'd left it last, under a stack of camouflage uniforms he'd taken from the last gang of traffickers. Nestled next to his bow was a quiver of his favorite recurve ammo: pencil-thin arrows with razor-sharp blades. He hauled up the lethal combo, then grabbed a cylinder of light red tarp.

"Let's hustle," Robert said. "We're running late."

Mel huffed behind as Robert and Armando wrangled through a vine-thick tangle behind the artillery hut; within minutes they all stopped on the edge of a large grassy expanse, studded with widely spaced thick-branched trees. A massive boar grazed about two football fields away.

"I don't see anything," Mel whispered. "And what's that cracking sound?"

"Macadamia nuts," Armando whispered back, handing Mel his field glasses.

"Shh." Robert dropped to one knee.

They hunkered down with him.

Robert remained silent. The boar looked up from its feeding, gave a cursory glance in their direction, then went back to crunching.

"Oh, now I see it!" Mel exclaimed.

"Shh!" Robert rasped. "God*damn*, Mel."

"Sorry," Mel whispered back. "But Robert, that thing is two city blocks away. Boars don't have super hearing, do they?"

"He knows we're here." Robert notched an arrow into his bow.

"You getting ready to shoot already?" Mel said. "Don't we have to figure out an approach first?"

"Robert is a very good archer," Armando said.

"Oh sure," Mel said. "Shoot him from here. No problem. Just tack a GPS on the arrow and type in, *humungous beast*."

"Not only am I going to shoot it from here," Robert whispered. "I'm going to shoot him in the midbrain."

"The foramen ovale?" Mel asked.

"And the medulla." Robert rose slowly. "Instant death. No nerve conduction between prefrontal cortex and limbic system. Heart and breathing stop. The beast won't feel a thing. A straight mercy shot." Robert steadied his breath as he pulled back the bow.

"Guillermo teaches us," Armando said in a church-soft voice, "that animals and people come from and return to what he calls the same generous nothing. We share the same parents and home. When the animal's time comes to feed us, we kill it with no pain, just as we would like to go when it is our time to feed the ground."

Armando's soothing voice helped calm Robert, and he began to feel one with the slight flowing breeze. He saw the lightly dancing leaves and swaying branches his arrow would have to traverse and let the breeze adjust his aim. His vision darted to the boar.

The cracking of the nutshells mixed with the rustling leaves and Robert's easy breathing. The rhythms filled the growing silence of Robert's focus.

As he waited for the boar to swallow again, Robert used his breathing to fine-tune his aim. The boar pulled back its lips and seemed to zoom right at Robert, who breathed out and freed the bowstring.

The arrow arced across the distance toward the boar, whose watchful eyes registered the last twenty yards of the incoming missile as calmly as if it were one of the huge dragonflies that festooned the area. Even from their distance, Robert and his cohorts could see the boar fall first on its front legs as if heaving up a final prayer, then slowly slump to its side, lifeless as a sculpture.

The group walked over to the spot.

"Feels like holy ground somehow," Mel said.

Robert looked over with surprise and approval. Mel's usual jaded expression had left his face entirely, replaced with a somber look that seemed to reveal the real Mel.

They reached the fallen animal, and Robert pointed at the arrow radiating from its head, then to the first star in the darkening sky. "See, Mel?"

Mel stooped and his eyes seemed to x-ray the boar's head. "Arrow through the midbrain," he said, as if dictating an autopsy report. "Crossing the left frontal-temporal junction to the foramen ovale." He looked up at Robert and nodded. "That's some kickass shot."

Robert nodded back, then leaned down and placed a hand on the animal's chest. Armando did the same. Mel's confusion turned to understanding, and he placed his hand by theirs, making a kind of finger and palm mandala over the beast's heart. All three bowed their heads in silence for a bit until Mel said in a prayerful voice, "And good eating, amen."

At this they all laughed and stood briskly.

Robert unrolled the tarp and placed it on the ground. Without being asked, Armando quickly field-dressed the beast, slicing open the skin of the belly and taking out the intestines and reproductive organs. As soon as he was done,

Mel helped him swing the obese animal onto the red sheet, which sank under the weight of the boar as they lifted it. The material was sturdy polypropylene, though, and they dragged the dinner safely back to the village.

All the villagers had gathered hungrily around Guillermo's fire, preparing and setting out dishes to accompany the kill: tamales wrapped in green maxan leaves, stuffed zucchini, pickled white fiambre salad, mole de platanos, and more.

There were no pleasantries at their arrival. People had confidence in Robert's hunting and expected him to bring home the bacon, no matter how monstrous. It was as normal to their life as takeout delivery in New York.

Guillermo's glare at Robert indicated they had exceeded their fifteen-minute deadline, but the medicine man didn't belabor it. Lately, Robert had been finding him edgier than usual. He suspected something unusual brewing in his mentor's deeper vision, some new concern for his people, who were always in his heart and mind.

Lingering pain from having to burn down their last village to ward off the narcotraficantes?

Robert thought about it then rejected this notion. His mentor wasn't one to dwell that way on the past. Guillermo's concerns were always about the present.

Was he worried about new attacks?

But the current village was nowhere near the major trails taking people to Kundal.

Something's eating him up, though, and knowing Guillermo, it's something real. Some new danger closing in on us.

A swarm of kids began butchering the carcass with fierce concentration, quickly passing large chunks of meat to the cooks, who waved their long-handled pans over the fire.

Soon loud sizzling and mouth-watering aromas filled the air, and the young butchers began singing a work song as they cut and sawed more meat from the boar.

Mel watched the communal process like a young boy mesmerized by the activity in a construction site. Robert clapped him on the back and said, "Let me show you to your hut, Mel."

Mel turned to him, startled out of his daze. "What? Oh! My hut. My five-star accommodations. Yes. You bet. I'm looking forward to a nice shower before dining."

"More like a small pan of greenish water."

"Figured as much. Listen, that'll do. I'm grateful for that much."

They approached a group of small, tidy structures.

"This hut's yours." Robert indicated one that looked like all the others. "My hut's right next to it, and Ernesto is your neighbor on the other side."

"Thanks, Robert." Mel gave him a squinting look. "There's a lot more to you than meets the eye."

"I guess."

Robert didn't want to get into it, but Mel pushed on. "And maybe there's a lot about you I *do* know," he paused for a moment, staring at Robert. "For example, all this jungle violence might explain why those cops, Macy and Landers, kept dropping by the ER, even weeks after you'd left, asking about you. Drilling that social worker about where you were. Asking me about your psychiatric history. About your mental state. Your checkered past. We all said nothing, of course, but Jesus, man—what kind of stuff were you involved in?"

"Nothing, Mel. Really."

"Wait a second ..." For a brief instant Mel's expression darkened. Then his face went ashen. "The kids from Atlanta, the ones murdered by those racists. The staff saw you storm out of the ER. You called in sick. I didn't hear from you until you showed up at my office a few days later. You were wounded."

"Mel, I don't want to talk about this now."

"Holy shit!" His expression suddenly brightened. "Are you the guy who took down that neo-Nazi group last winter? Are you the Manhattan Vigilante? The Prince of Payback?"

A triumphant smile tugged slightly at the corners of Robert's lips. "Is *The New York Post* still writing about me?"

"Of course!" The edges around Mel's eyes crinkled. "In fact, everyone is wondering where the hell you disappeared. There's some serial rapist named the Owl ravaging New York City, and you're the only thing they seem to want to write about."

"Seriously?" Robert asked.

"I knew that's why those cops were coming around so often, why they were asking the staff if you ever got violent."

"Listen, Mel, you have to promise me you won't say a word to anyone about this. I can get arrested and put away for a very long time if the cops find out. Let's drop the subject and move on."

"I understand." They stared at each other a few beats, then Mel nodded. "Enough said. Let me wash the pig schmutz off me before our pork chops. I'm glad I don't keep kosher."

CHAPTER 7

Robert's favorite part of jungle life was dinner. Not only the freshness of the food served so beautifully on long wooden platters, but also how it recharged the communal energy. Everyone fed each other's spirit like the food fed their bodies. Robert had dreaded his meals in New York, almost always eating alone or on the go. He blamed it on his dual life of manic ER doctor and maniac vigilante—but in the middle of the night, when he couldn't sleep, he knew better.

The price of being a loner is loneliness.

But Sharon had changed all that. She'd opened something in him that had long been shut. She saw his potential for goodness. Her optimism was refreshing. Being good and doing the right thing came naturally to her. That's what a doctor was supposed to do, but for Robert it was never that simple.

Here, with his new Guatemalan community surrounded not by walls but by the forest, sharing hearty meals and company, uplifted by the smiles and fire-lit faces animating the jungle night, he felt the strands of belonging wrap itself around him. This was his new home, with these people. Not an outside protector removed from his daily life, but someone who would do anything to protect them because they were his family.

My new family.

The ten-year-old boy who could run faster than any adult, whose prowess with the makeshift soccer ball would make any *fútbol* scout drool.

The young mother of six, who seemed to get more energy with each child she produced.

The rotund teacher, who every night sat before his hut talking with whoever stopped to sit about whatever came into his mind: from simple things, like what wood burns the cleanest, to big thoughts, like how to understand the passage of time.

Then there was the group of five males just beginning to grow facial hair, who seemed to always be getting into fights, wrestling matches that never led to serious injuries or broken friendships. The best-friend pair of keen-eyed adolescent girls who seemed to take in everything going on, with a politeness and respect that made them seem like fifty-year-old leaders. The crone with her huge one-tooth smile. The drummer with the crazy eyes who could start his mesmerizing rhythms any time of day or night. The poor, tormented graybeard with withered arms and legs, who couldn't finish any sentence he started. The babies, the toddlers, the young children—their emerging personalities one of the things most talked about around the late-night fire. The muscular Miguel, who read every printed thing he could find, who had volumes of ratty paper filled with writing he penned at night by candlelight and wouldn't show anyone.

And Armando, sunken-chested but strong like steel cable, savvy and itching for action with a hard glint of humor always in his eyes—permanently ready, it seemed, to either cut you down or make you laugh.

Robert could name every villager even from a far distance just by how they moved. He also found he talked and acted a bit differently with each person, a constant surprise that made him wonder how he had managed all his years with his gruff bedside manner and poor social skills. He shook his head thinking of how he and most people lived such separate lives in the U.S. and other Western countries. It helped explain why as a New York doctor he had run into so many cases of depression, and why he himself had woken so many mornings feeling like he couldn't go on living another day.

Families scattered all over the country. Community rare as diamonds and just as hard to form.

"I'm definitely feeling refreshed." Mel now sported a dry white shirt. "I splashed some of that green water on my face. As good as any shower I've ever taken."

"Here you go, boss." Robert handed Mel a plate of food heaped with boar meat, several steaming jungle greens mixed with nuts and coconut flakes, a colorful tamale and juicy slices of mango, avocado, and tomato.

"Mm." Mel bent to breathe in the plate's aromas. "I think this place could easily become my favorite restaurant. Thank you, Robert."

"Before you eat, though," Robert said, "drink this." He handed him a small wooden cup. Inside was a milky liquid.

Mel lifted the cup closer to his face and inspected it. He placed it close to his nose. "What the hell is it?"

"Nature's Gatorade. You're likely electrolyte depleted. You've been sweating like ten pigs and not replenishing. This drink will prevent cramps, headaches, fatigue, myositis."

Mel brought the liquid close to his face. Smelled it and shrugged. Then he drank it down in one long gulp. "Hmm! Not half-bad. What is it?"

"Semen we drained from the boar's scrotum. Lots of nutrients."

Mel started spitting and bent over, clutching his stomach. Miguel, who had overheard the exchange, laughed and came over and started patting Mel's back. "Mm, good pig juice!"

Other villagers heard and started laughing, too.

"I'll tell you a secret, Mel," Robert said, when Mel had stopped retching.

"What's that?" Mel wiped his mouth and groaned.

"That was really just coconut juice with some citrus and salt thrown in."

"You bastard!"

Robert, Miguel, and several others nearby burst into laughter. Mel looked around. A smile of delighted amusement played on his lips. He took a grand theatrical bow and received loud applause and some roars of approval. The drummer began rat-tat-tatting his wooden plate with his wooden spoons, creating an infectious rhythm that others picked up. The flirty young girls began dancing. Mel beamed with enjoyment, then sat and started to devour his dinner.

The drumming and dancing continued for a short while, then cross-faded into the waves of chatter and laughter that rose and fell around the fire like the flames themselves. The only person untouched by the festive mood was Guillermo, who stood apart from the fire with his arms crossed, pensive and not eating.

"What's up with him?" Mel asked.

"It's hard to describe," Robert said. "I think what he's doing is looking ten directions into the future of this village and not liking any path he sees."

"Interesting." Mel gnawed his way around a hambone. "I thought he was just pissed because we didn't make his deadline."

"There's something major going on in this jungle. Dark stuff. Some new evil worse than anything we've ever seen. He feels it. The man is cursed with a sixth sense. He knows evil lurks around us, and he has a sense of deep responsibility. He fears for his people, and when he fears, I do, too. I've never known anyone with such an accurate intuition."

Mel put down his cleaned plate with a thunk. "Now *I'm* worried."

"The more he stands there, the more his vibes get to me." Robert put down his half-filled plate. He looked across the fire, and Guillermo suddenly moved his head for the first time in five minutes, meeting Robert's eyes.

"Can he hear us?" Mel whispered.

Robert nodded at Guillermo, and Guillermo nodded back and looked into the distance again.

"Are you going to finish that?" Mel asked, pointing to Robert's plate.

"Feel free." Robert stared at his teacher. Guillermo's nod had extinguished what little appetite Robert had left.

"So what's going on, you think?" Mel snaked Robert's plate into his lap. "In the jungle. What dark stuff?"

"We haven't been able to figure it out yet." Robert picked out a stiff pine bristle from the ground to use as a toothpick. "But something rotten is going on. There's been an increase in drug trafficking around here. More than normal. But that's not it. There's been more kidnapping and human trafficking. Before, that was confined to the city. So why has it moved into this part of the jungle? It doesn't make sense. We've been able to ward off the traffickers so far, but for how long?"

"Can't the Guatemalan government help?"

"We've made requests. All ignored."

"Corruption?"

"Some corruption, yeah. And whatever else. Lack of interest and resources, maybe."

Mel was silent for a while. He put down his second cleaned plate and gave Robert a serious look. "How did you get involved in all this? You're a doctor, and it sounds like what they need is a guerilla. You should stick to fighting diseases, not bad guys."

Mel's words made Robert think of Sharon and all the arguments he'd had with her about his double life. That life he thought he'd left behind had followed him deep into Guatemala. "I learned I could fight both diseases and bad guys from Guillermo over there. I met him fifteen years ago when I rotated down here during medical school. Back then, there was a civil war. He taught me medicine and warfare. Guillermo is a master of both."

Mel cast his gaze across the high-dancing flames at Guillermo's ramrod figure. "I can tell. I know he's a lot older than I am, but he looks thirty years younger. I definitely would not want to fuck with him in a fight."

"No one would," Robert said. "But hey, you're not here for long, right? Let's get back to Francine. Where are her medical records?"

Mel pulled the thick manila folder from the bag at his feet. "Here's everything."

As Robert browsed through the paperwork, his eyes burned with a mixture of alertness and excitement. It'd been over two months since he'd looked at blood results and imaging studies. He was surprised to find his fingers tingling with pleasure as he turned the pages.

Still, Robert knew full well he preferred travel medicine, doctoring on the go, dealing with patients in their natural environment. Even with limited resources, medicine in the jungle fired up every doctor nerve in his body. Diagnosing solely by giving a physical exam and extracting the patient's history aroused his greatest gifts as a physician. Direct doctor-patient interchange was the foundation of all healing, but most of the medical community these days seemed to be doing it less and less. With the availability of blood tests as well as CT, MRI, and other imaging studies, medical students and residents relied more on technology than old-school hands-on physician attention.

Robert had lost almost all patience with the whole hospital system. Patients were parked in closed-off buildings. Confined to a bed. No open-window ventilation. No exercise or time in nature.

No wonder thousands of patients die every year in hospitals. They get sicker, not healthier.

Robert looked around, marveling at the beauty of the great outdoors around him. The rich, humid air seemed to nourish him with every breath. The rhythms and sounds of the forest were music to his ears, unlike the artificial beepings and clacks that punctured a hospital's atmosphere.

What would happen if patients had an opportunity to heal somewhere open to the sensations of nature?

He looked back at the pile of papers in his hands and riffled through them. "You weren't joking about a full workup."

"Nothing she didn't get, no one who didn't take a shot. Neurology, cardiology, rheumatology. Valentine even got infectious disease on board. Then he had the interventional radiologist perform a lumbar puncture. More tests, more scans, cardiac panel, rheumatological studies—nothing! Might as well have just asked a Ouija board. The more labs we got back, the more confused we all grew—and the more I regretted letting you go. Thank God Reede put me onto your whereabouts."

Robert squared up the papers. "You know what, Mel? Once we crack this, I might just take you up on your offer of my old job."

Mel's face perked up.

"You'd have to talk the board into it, though. Kiss a lot of weasel ass."

"I'll do that and more."

Armando emerged before them as if he'd dropped from the night sky. "Roberto, we have a problem."

CHAPTER 8

"*Que pasa?*" Robert sprang to his feet.

"Narcotraficantes." Armando spat angrily. "Whole new group."

"How many this time?" Robert asked.

"Eight men, six hostages."

Guillermo appeared behind Armando's shoulder. "Gear up, Roberto. Let's go."

Robert ran to his hut and began to lock and load, his hatred of traffickers making his blood boil.

The story was far too common. Girls kidnapped and raped and beaten and sold as prostitutes, forced to perform sex acts all day and night for years. Decimated by syphilis, herpes, HPV, gonorrhea, chlamydia, and HIV. Then thrown away like garbage in their thirties—into homelessness and wretchedness.

Robert trotted back to Guillermo with tight fists, thinking maybe he wouldn't go back to New York City after all.

Mel came panting up to them. "I'm going with you guys."

Guillermo slammed his spear into the ground so hard it made sparks fly up from the fire. He growled to Robert. "Please tell your former boss we don't need him snapping branches and huffing like a gutted bear while we sneak up on these terrorists, who would shove a stick through his asshole and out his mouth and barbecue him over an open fire all night for their next day's breakfast."

"That's a little harsh," Mel said weakly, looking pale.

Robert gently patted Mel in the back. "It's okay, boss. Thanks for offering. It's better if you hang back here in camp. We got this. When I get back I'll get to Francine's records and have an answer for you by morning. Get some rest. You'll need it. It's a long hike back to Guatemala City."

"Come on, Robert. How can just three of you take on eight guys? And with hostages?"

"Only two of us," Guillermo said.

"No, way!" Armando shot back. "I'm going too. I spotted them."

"No," Guillermo said, his face as hard and expressionless as a skull. "You're still a cub."

"Not any more, Father! I've done everything you've asked of me. I've trained enough. I'm ready."

Mel's eyes had grown wide. Robert knew he was surprised to realize Guillermo had such a young son.

He'd be even more shocked to learn that Guillermo's ex-wife was Rivera, his triage nurse in New York.

"I've already spoken." Guillermo's commanding voice made Armando take a step back. Robert could see he was seething but savvy enough to stay mute. Once Guillermo made a decision, it became law. There was no going against it.

"Soon, Armando." Robert squeezed his shoulder. "Your time to be a hero is coming. I know it as well as I know you."

Armando shrugged off Robert's hand and stormed away to his hut.

"He's very close to ready, Guillermo."

"An arrow that's close to hitting a target does no one any good. It only makes the enemy madder. He's not ready."

Guillermo wrapped a quiver heavy with arrows around his tightly packed body. "He's quick as a snake, his marksmanship is superb, but he hasn't balanced his thinking yet. It's still more playful than serious."

"And he's your son and you don't want him getting hurt."

Guillermo glared at Robert.

Robert kept his mouth shut. He'd made his point and pushed it as far as he could.

"Seriously, guys," Mel interrupted. "How do you Rambos expect to rescue those girls? Two against eight?"

Robert turned away from Guillermo, grateful for the interruption. "Don't worry, Mel. We've gone against way more than eight and we're still here."

"You're crazy. You're a doctor not a Navy SEAL."

"When you get home there's a book you can read that can help explain it. *The Art of War* by Sun Tzu."

"I read that book in college. It improved my poker winnings but that's about it." Mel's voice dropped an octave and his face turned pale. "You guys are going after armed drug guerillas. You think bows and arrows are going to help? Are you going to shoot their water bottles out of their hands like you did mine?"

"We'll do a bit more than that." Robert smiled. "I'm going to hunt these guys down like the boar, but I won't be as gentle."

CHAPTER 9

Robert and Guillermo lay on their bellies, peering down from a hill at the shadowy procession below. The half-moon lent a ghostly aura to the cruel march, and the faint whimpers from the young hostages mixed with their sad shuffling. Robert spied six stumbling girls with handcuffs at the wrists linked by a long metal chain that picked up glints of moonlight.

Two groups of four men in camouflage flanked the girls and prodded them with military assault rifles. If Robert's glare could kill, all eight would be instantly decapitated, their heads thudding on the jungle floor like so many coconuts swollen with larvae.

His fury at the sight pumped his heart into overdrive. His fingers began to twitch, and Guillermo pressed a calming hand between his shoulder blades.

Somehow this stopped the tremor and cooled the fire in Robert's chest.

They both stood and headed quickly toward the caravan's next turn. They slipped across the crest of the hill as quiet as the slight breeze riffling the grass beneath them.

The sexual slave trade had been blighting humanity for centuries, but only recently had it invaded Guatemala—probably because of the spreading drug plague.

For the last two years, Guillermo had been trying to dig up the name of the operation's honcho. Every lamebrain narcotraficante they caught he'd interrogate mercilessly, but no one knew or would tell—even after harsh solitary confinement in cramped makeshift prisons.

Robert was on board with Guillermo in doing everything they could to find the guy's identity. The head of this operation had to be found and killed. Too many lives were being shattered.

Things have changed so much since I was last here. This incredible jungle! Now filling with everything ugly and crass.

Guatemala City polluted with choking air and political corruption. Not what I was expecting when I left New York.

Robert's plan had been to return here and heal in the wide arms of the jungle. To settle and center himself, to let the peace of its sunrise and the serenity of its starlit nights end the war he felt tearing his insides apart.

To get the psychological rest he needed to return to Sharon as the man she always saw in him.

A wave of guilt traveled through Robert's gut. He was failing miserably at that goal. Sharon would hate what he was about to do. She wanted no part of him as a vigilante.

Wouldn't she hate even more the violence the narcotraficantes were inflicting on these girls?

They came to the ridge overlying the turn. Above their slight panting, they could hear the faintest sounds of the approaching slave march.

"Plan?" Robert whispered, trying to push Sharon-thoughts from his mind. He needed to be on full alert.

"They're too close to the hostages to take from here." Guillermo studied the emerging human train.

He was right. Their arrows could down some of the guards right away, but in the melee that would follow, the hostages would be in too much danger.

Too much crossfire.

"So?" Robert looked expectantly at his mentor.

Guillermo stared back evenly. "You tell me."

Robert gazed back down. The group would come directly below them very shortly. He pored over his knowledge of military strategy from the dozens of books in his head and the thousands of hours he'd spent with Guillermo.

What technique would work best in this situation?

"Distraction," Robert whispered.

"What else?" Guillermo shook his head in disapproval. "You better start focusing or we're going to end up dead."

Robert blinked as Guillermo's words stung him.

He's right. Sharon is getting in the way.

"Become one with the enemy," Robert whispered, the thought coming into his head as soon as he shook Sharon out of it. "Infiltrate the group."

Guillermo nodded, his eyes as dangerous as a burning fuse. "Go now. We have less than a minute to intercept them."

CHAPTER 10

"Help! Please, somebody help. Where is everyone? Where'd you all go?"

Robert yelled at the top of his lungs when the group of hostages and narcos made the turn and saw him. He acted terrified. He had messed up his hair, taken his shirt off, wrapped it around his waist, and rubbed dirt into his torso and face.

Suddenly eight guns were aimed at him. He felt his heartbeat thrumming in his neck. He knew these thugs would shoot him without asking questions. He was banking on their surprise and desire for information about anyone else in the area.

"Please!" Robert reached for the sky. "Don't shoot!" he yelled again, his voice quivering with fright.

"Who the fuck are you?" demanded a bushy-bearded squat man, stepping forward.

The leader. He goes first. Cocky little shitbag with a Napoleon complex.

"My name is Daniel Crawford," Robert blustered in an anxious rush. "I'm here with a tour group. We're hiking up to Kundal. I just had to pee bad, you know, too many *cervezas* last night, and something bit me and I yelled and ran and next thing I know I lost my group." Robert buried his head in his hands and made sobbing noises. No tears, though, filled his eyes, which were hot and dry with intent and calculation.

Narcos are still too close to the girls.

He heard them arguing in vulgar Spanish.

Robert spat into his hands and lifted his head from them, wiping at his eyes, smearing saliva on his cheeks to look like tears. Squat Beard was still eyeing him while jawing with another little bearded guy who looked like a brother or cousin. They were still too close to the hostages. Robert had to get them to move before Guillermo could start the carnage.

"Kundal is closed, you white piece of shit," the leader crowed. "You and your group should know that. There are signs all over. I think you're too dumb to live. What do you say, amigos? Too dumb to live?"

His troop cheered and laughed, and the petty tyrant puffed his chest out in pleasure.

"I may be dumb but I love your country," Robert whined. "The others do, too. We're crazy about Mayan culture and came here dying to see Kundal. Please, amigo! When my friends and I learned Kundal was closed, we vowed to sneak into the ruins if we had to. Our plane tickets were nonrefundable."

"How many of you are there?" the leader asked.

"Six … plus a guide. A huge man. A bear!" Robert had to struggle to keep a straight face.

"Six plus one," the leader yelled, and again his men let loose their fawning laughter. Then he turned again to his weak-chinned brother and they bickered about what to do. If they shot Robert, the noise might bring the others and the bear around. Or it might make the bear phone troublesome authorities. Maybe they should cut Robert's throat—not as much noise. Or send four of them out to hunt down the other tourists and cut their throats, too. Robert sensed that Americans heading for the ruins troubled them.

The men weren't moving from their shielded position behind the cluster of dull-eyed hostages. Robert had to try something else.

He took a couple of steps to the side and put his hands in his pocket. "I have gold. Lots of gold. *Mucho oro*! We found a chest of coins under the high roots of a great Ceiba tree. Look, I have some!" He put both hands under his waist-draped shirt as if to pull coins from his pocket.

The leader and his brother stepped closer to look and immediately Robert heard a double thrum growing louder. The fake fear on his face instantly turned into a sigh of elation.

One arrow tore through the leader's jugular, his hands flying to his neck as he collapsed, while the other drove through his brother's left eye and into the brain, killing him before he hit the group. Guillermo had double-strung two arrows and shot them with a sniper's accuracy.

Two guards were now raising their rifles behind the fallen leaders. In one smooth motion, each of Robert's hands pulled out an FGX Jungle Dart knife and sent their dusky blades deep into the nerves of their bellies, paralyzing them instantly. Before they had time to fall, Robert scrambled forward and ripped their guns from their jerking fingers, and turned. A tall man dashed toward him with a karate yell he must have learned from a kung fu movie. Snarling, Robert stepped forward and jabbed the barrel of the rifle into his howling mouth and pulled the trigger, showering the bushes behind him with brains and dark blood that glistened where the pale light struck it.

Most of the girls were coming to life now. A few screamed as two more simultaneous arrows pierced the sternum of one guard and the green bandana covering the larynx of another. As they gurgled and tried in vain to pull the arrows out, the last remaining guard started to run into the forest, but one raven-haired girl with the musculature of a healthy farm worker tripped him. He cursed and tried to strike her as he rose to his feet, but Robert caught the man's fist and squeezed, hearing the crack of breaking knuckles under the man's screams. Then the girl took one bounding step and kicked the guy's groin hard enough to silence him, his mouth a startled O. Robert knocked him unconscious with a lightning elbow to his ear.

The whole thing took less than a minute.

"Keep those you can alive," he heard Guillermo yelling, running down the hill. "We'll get them to talk."

A second later the din of automatic fire exploded through the air. Robert whirled and groaned. The farm girl had emptied the guard's automatic rifle into his genitals, and now spat on him and screamed close into his face as the light went out of his eyes:

"Violador! Asesino! Hijo de puta!"

Rapist! Murderer! Son of a bitch!

A few of the other girls cheered their blood-curdling approval and came over and spat on the man and kicked dirt on what was left of him.

Then all the life seemed to go out of the girls. They sat, some trembling, some whimpering, some keening a high-pitched sound. The brawny farm girl began checking each one of them, comforting them as best she could.

Some leaders are born out of tragedy.

Robert ripped the pockets off the head narco until he found the key to the handcuffs. He began releasing the girls, murmuring gentle words to them.

The adrenaline from the code-red action had him taking deep breaths to stop his knees and hands from shaking. He heard the guard with the arrow through his throat still gurgling, but a quick glance told him the young idiot was not far from bleeding out.

Guillermo arrived a few minutes later, a bit out of breath from the hike down. Some of the girls gave startled yelps at the fearsome armed man, but he quickly dropped his bow and calmed them with his grandfatherly voice. "It's all right, *chicas.* It's all over. We'll take you to your village in the morning. Tonight you'll come to our village, get food and rest …"

The guard with the arrow in his throat had not moved since Guillermo arrived, but now suddenly made an awful drowning sound, and his eyes shot open in terror as if the stars were falling on him like glowing demons coming to take him to hell. Guillermo glanced over at the sound and his brown face drained, resembling in profile the half-moon itself, dotted with a blinking eye.

He leapt toward the writhing kid like a wildcat at a scurrying rodent. "What are you doing here? Who sent you?" he yelled. "Who are you working for?" Guillermo was almost incoherent with rage. "Talk to me!"

"*Perdon, tio …*" the boy rasped.

And then he went limp.

The shouting had silenced all the girls.

Robert called to him. "Guillermo? Are you okay?"

Without looking back, Guillermo swept up his bow and rushed off toward the village.

CHAPTER 11

As soon as Robert led the exhausted girls into the village, people began emerging with food and water and caring expressions. Robert proceeded straight to Guillermo's hut. At the doorway, Armando was asking his father if he could enter, and Guillermo kept barking at him to go away. When Armando saw Robert, he rushed to him and asked how it had gone. Robert told him of the diversion, Guillermo's double-arrow shots …

"I can do that same shot," Armando interrupted excitedly. "I worked on it yesterday. Three out of five double hits!"

"That's great, Armando," Robert said. "You want to hear what happened, or are you angling for a training medal? Stop acting like a kid if you want to join a mission."

Armando looked startled.

Robert regretted the words as soon as they came out. But he realized then that Guillermo was right.

Armando wasn't ready.

"Come on." Robert put a hand on Armando's shoulder. "I'll take you in to see your father. He'll tell you what you can do to help."

Armando swallowed and nodded. "Yes, sir."

Robert whacked him gently on the back of his head, and they entered the hut.

Guillermo looked up fiercely. "Get him out of here!"

Armando stepped forward. "Tell me how I can help, Father, and I'll go."

Guillermo marched right up to Armando and looked into his eyes, checking out his manner. Armando gazed right back, the way Robert had looked at him a minute ago.

"Go set up sleeping places for the girls," Guillermo said finally, and walked over to the one chair in the hut and sat. "Have Yolanda help clean them up and see that they're fed and warm. Tomorrow you and Miguel will take them back to their village."

"I'll get it done." Armando left briskly to carry out the orders.

Guillermo sat looking at the doorway as if his son were still there. Robert saw a smile flicker on his lips, wiped immediately away by a sigh and a faint trace of grief and anger.

"Are you going to tell me what's going on?" Robert asked.

Guillermo sighed again. "That kid I shot."

"With the green bandana?"

Guillermo nodded. "I knew him. One of my former students."

"Oh. Sorry, Guillermo. That's hard."

"He was my friend's kid. My best friend. The boy wanted to be a physician, he wanted to make his father proud. To save his life. My friend had real bad kidneys. He had three sons. Manuel was the youngest. We called him Manny, the little devil. He was a handful but dead set on sucking up everything he could about medicine. I took him under my wing, him and his brothers, taught them everything I could about tropical medicine and doctoring. We'd go on long hikes collecting herbs. That's how Manny learned to navigate these parts." Guillermo grew silent as a bitter look settled into his face.

"This before I came here for my med school rotation?"

"A few years before." Guillermo came out of his daze. "The brothers were already going on house calls with me. But then their father died of renal failure and their mother moved them to Guatemala City. I hadn't heard from them in all these years. But it was Manny. I know it. How could I forget that kid?"

Although Guillermo's grief was deep and heart wrenching, tears were nowhere near his eyes.

"You had no choice," Robert said.

"I realize that."

"Plus, you saved my life."

"I know." Guillermo went to the doorway, spat, and came back in, rubbing his face. "Trafficking girls? What the hell happened to him?"

"It's been years since you saw him. People change. Drugs. Money problems. Extortion. Who knows?"

"What's happening to our country, Robert? It's falling down a shit pit and we can't do anything to stop it."

"We're doing what we can."

There was a brief silence as Guillermo sat down again. He heaved a sigh. "You ever wonder if it's all a myth?"

"What's that?" Robert asked.

"Good beating out evil." Guillermo's eyes stared right at Robert.

"Of course," Robert said. "The bad guys don't play by our rules. That's why we decided we would ignore them, too. But we're only two people, and there's an army of evil out there."

Guillermo nodded solemnly.

"Knock, knock," Mel said in the doorway, then stepped in. "What happened out there?"

"Not now," Robert said. "Go get some sleep. I'll get to Francine's report in a bit and get back to you in the morning."

"I don't expect to be sleeping for a while, Robert. Those girls need medical attention. They're all traumatized to some extent, and not just by the traffickers."

"What is he talking about?" Guillermo snapped.

"I'm talking about what they just saw. The carnage." Mel took a couple of steps closer. "Did you guys really just slaughter those young men? I'm asking respectfully."

"He's asking *respectfully*?" Guillermo said to Robert, his voice dripping with venom.

"We were protecting the girls from death, Mel, or something worse."

"I know you told me to drop the subject, but now I feel I need to say what's on my mind." Mel's eyes narrowed just slightly. "While I'm in awe that you singlehandedly took down the Aryan brotherhood in Manhattan, I'm shocked you got involved in that kind of activity in the first place. I thought we were doctors, Robert. And you too, Guillermo. Life is sacred and all that good stuff. Last time I looked, the Hippocratic Oath didn't say anything about going on a killing spree."

"In my hut, the air is mine!" Guillermo snapped. "Get that wheezer out of here, Robert, or I'll make sure he gets a taste of solitary confinement."

Robert tugged Mel to the doorway and spoke low and hard. "There's too much about me and what goes on in this jungle you don't know, Mel. So get your ass off your high horse before you break its back."

They stepped outside. The night air was thick with humidity, and the bugs and night critters were almost as loud as the traffic in midtown Manhattan.

"How can I drop it, Robert? I mean, I may know far from everything about you and your mentor over there, but how can I give you back your old job at St. Jude's knowing you like to take an after-dinner walk, go slay some bad guys, then come back to have a fun little bull session with your co-felon. You guys could go to jail for this! And I could be arrested as an accessory."

"There is no danger of that," Guillermo snapped, approaching Mel.

Robert took a step back. Mel had been warned. He had Guillermo to deal with now.

"Look," Mel said to the medicine man. "I get it. I'm not stupid. Those eight guys at the very least facilitated brutal kidnapping, torture, rape, and probably murder. But you're not judge and jury. They needed to be arrested. They needed a trial. Then maybe the electric chair could malfunction and fry them for a few hours until their blood turned to steam and their heads popped off like whistling fireworks—whatever. I get it. But this? Makes you so-called healers seem too much like the psycho scum you're trying to rub out."

"The police and judges here are as bad as the scum," Guillermo shot back, taking his knife out and pointing it at Mel. "You don't know anything about my country. We are all our people have, and all your bullshit talk does them as much good as a bag of Doritos. Imagine you're Francine, your dear wife who's gone into a coma, no doubt to get away from your reeking mound of bullshit." Guillermo now advanced the knife on Mel until its point touched his neck. "That's right, you're Francine and I'm the poor innocent-until-proven-guilty terrorist kid ready to rape you at knife point. And her lousy, useless husband is tied to that chair over there watching." He dragged the knife down over Mel's quivering torso. "And Robert here bursts into the room waving an arrest warrant. How's that sound, Dr. Weiss? What do you think would happen? You like that scenario? Or how about Robert puts an arrow through my eye and saves your wife's life? Which scenario would you choose, you righteous asshole?"

"Easy, Guillermo." Robert stepped forward and eased the knife away from Mel's sweat-drenched body. "Enough already. He has no experience with this."

"It's time he got his cherry popped, don't you think? You liberal Americans, blind to the realities of human nature." Guillermo whirled on Robert. "And what's happened to you? I was going to keep my mouth shut, but you've changed since New York. That new girl, I bet. That goddamn Sharon."

Robert winced to hear her name spoken so sourly.

"I knew it," Guillermo went on. "It *is* her! A woman? You let a woman take your edge away? In this jungle, with things so dire. That's why you want to leave me? Leave us all?"

"I'm here because I want to be, and you know it," Robert protested.

"Your voice has cracks in it," Guillermo shot back.

They stood jaw to jaw, breathing in each other's air, each searching the other's eyes for how much they could trust each other now.

"I came here on my own terms, Guillermo," Robert finally said, "and I'll stay as long as you need me. You are my real father, and everyone here is my family."

There was an uncomfortable silence, then Guillermo's tense shoulders relaxed and lowered. "I can tell you mean that, but I know your thoughts go back to her more and more. Soon you'll be useless here. You can't be in two places at once. You should go back with your former boss tomorrow. I'll blow these bastards out of this jungle on my own or end up in the jungle upstairs, drinking beer, looking down and wondering why the hell I cared so much about this moldy crumb of a planet."

Robert didn't respond. He stared into the forest, wondering what to do.

Mel had finished wiping his sweaty face with the bottom of his shirt, and jumped to Robert's defense. "If Robert says he'll hang with you, he will. Maybe you need him around to temper how crazy violent you get, sticking a knife at my throat. I'm the farthest thing from an enemy you'll ever meet."

"It's not my problem you can't play a little rough." Guillermo slid the knife back into the sheath at his hip.

"I don't appreciate being treated like a psychopath by someone whose eyes are rolling around in his head. Who are you to decide who deserves execution?"

Again Guillermo got in Mel's face, his mood springing from jocular to tigerish in an instant. "I know who deserves waking up, and I know who deserves killing."

"That's the truth, Mel," Robert said. "Without Guillermo we'd all be buzzard lunch."

"I'll tell you what's true about me," Mel said, not backing away an inch. "I could never kill someone. It doesn't matter what they've done ..."

At that moment Armando burst in.

"We need a doctor! One of the girls is dying."

CHAPTER 12

They found the girl on the ground, surrounded by anxious villagers and tearful friends. She was about thirteen, in ragged jeans and a yellow T-shirt, her long brown hair in pigtails. She held her hands scared stiff at her right side. Her sweat-slick face was ashen, and she winced with pain.

"*Que te pasa?*" Robert asked as he knelt over the girl.

"Hurts," she rasped, blinking back tears.

"You stay brave," Mel said gently, kneeling to join Robert. "We're going to help. What's your name?"

"Maria," she whispered.

"Beautiful name," Mel said. "Like the cool stars shining down now. You see them?'

"*S-s-si.*" She turned her eyes skyward. The distraction of serene nature seemed to ease her for a moment.

Robert meanwhile had been speeding through the diagnostic checklist he first learned in his emergency medicine rotation in medical school.

Three questions.

One: Is the patient sick?

Two: What are the vital signs?

Three: What is the differential diagnosis of the patient's complaint?

Answer to question one was obvious. The patient was hunched, perspiring, and in acute distress.

She's sick.

"According to her friends," Armando began, "she's been complaining of stomach cramps the past three days. The right side. She was beaten and gang-raped before they started marching, and she hasn't eaten since—but she vomited twice before you guys rescued her and once after."

"Thanks, Armando," Robert said.

Vital signs.

Robert took the girl's wrist, placed two fingers on top of her radial artery and started counting.

Pulse weak but palpable. Heart rate one-hundred-forty.

She was cold and clammy.

Respiratory rate … thirty.

He pulled her lower eyelid down. Her conjunctiva was pink, which meant there was no anemia. He felt her abdomen. She grimaced and flailed her hands at his.

Guarding. Severely tender. Mild rebound.

Blood pressure low, heart rate up. Right lower quadrant pain.

Could be a hundred things: kidney stone, pyelonephritis, ovarian cyst or torsion, tubo-ovarian abscess.

But top on the differential: ectopic pregnancy or appendicitis.

Best guess for a girl this young, recently gang-raped …

Ectopic pregnancy.

"Are you thinking what I'm thinking?" Guillermo wiped the girl's face with a damp cloth that smelled of lemon and mint.

"Ectopic," Mel whispered.

"Yeah," Robert said, knowing all three of them understood the need to make sure the girl didn't have a tubal pregnancy. "Let's get her to the infirmary there." He indicated with his chin a spreading tent with large open windows twenty yards away.

They lifted the girl carefully and carried her into the tent; the whole time Mel told her what a special young woman she was, how she was being so brave.

After they lowered her onto a stretcher bed, Guillermo examined her in half the time it had taken Robert. "Start an IV," he said. "We need a pregnancy test."

"You guys have pregnancy tests?" Mel asked.

"Of course." Robert opened a cabinet stacked with antibiotics, pain medications, IV fluids—all sorts of supplies that Guillermo and Robert had garnered from Guatemala City, not to mention the mother lode Robert had "borrowed" from the St. Jude's ER storage room and shipped to Guatemala right before he left New York.

Mel gaped at the supplies as Robert extracted a sealed package. "You'd be surprised what we got," Robert said. "No ultrasound, though."

"It might not be an ectopic," Guillermo said, "but let's check first."

"It could be appendicitis," Robert said.

"What if it's an ectopic?" Mel asked.

"Either way, we need to transport her to Guatemala City," Robert said. "Any surgical or tough OB/GYN cases go there."

"Culdocentesis would show a ruptured ectopic," Mel mused, then shook his head. "But she'd have to rupture."

"Ready to hydrate." Guillermo bent to the girl. "Maria," he said, "first we need you to urinate some so we can test what's wrong with you."

The girl's eyes widened and she shook her head rapidly back and forth, her breath verging on panic. Guillermo quickly backed away and beckoned for Yolanda, the young mother of six, to come over. "Get some urine from her." He handed her a sample cup.

"Okay." Yolanda took the cup, knelt, smoothed Maria's hair, and murmured gently to her. Maria's breathing calmed. Then the fear drained from her eyes and she squeezed them tight. When they opened after a while, they were full of tears.

"I can't, " she said weakly. "I'm sorry."

"Shh," Yolanda cooed, putting the back of her hand on the girl's cheek. "It's all right, it's okay. Take your time."

"No, it's not okay," Guillermo grumbled under his breath. "She has to squeeze out a few drops. Otherwise, we place a Foley and straight catheterize her bladder."

"Get a little blood from her IV," Mel said. "Use it instead of the urine for the test."

"What are you talking about?" Guillermo snapped.

"There was a study out of Maimonides Hospital in New York. You can use blood to test for pregnancy. The test picks up the beta hCG in the blood better than it does in the urine."

"I've never heard of that," Guillermo said.

"I have," Robert said. "The study has been confirmed. Good sensitivity, especially for ectopic."

Guillermo growled and pulled a milliliter of blood from the girl's IV prior to starting her on the fluids. Then he placed several drops on the pregnancy strip and held it out.

A minute later it was confirmed. She was not pregnant.

"I still wouldn't trust that," Guillermo said. "Think about it. She's been raped. She has severe abdominal pain. She's guarding. It's an ectopic until proven otherwise."

"I hate to disagree with you," Robert said, "but I'm confident that the test is sensitive enough to rule out an ectopic. We have to assume she's not pregnant and work from there."

Guillermo didn't say anything.

"Okay," Mel said, "What do we do now?"

Robert grew pensive. "It could still be pelvic, but it's likely appendicitis. We need to transfer her."

"Bad idea," Mel said. "Look at her." Maria's grimacing face was now perspiring more than ever. Despite Yolanda's tender ministrations, her gaze was looking further and further into the distance. "That's bad sepsis. The appendix is about to rupture or maybe it already has. Any delay now could kill her."

"We can start her on IV antibiotics," Robert said. "That'll buy us some time ..."

"We can do the surgery here." Mel's voice was filled with conviction. He walked to the supplies, pulled out a scalpel, a sterile gown, gloves, and several syringes.

"Hey," Guillermo hissed. "No cowboy medicine in my tent! I haven't done an appendectomy in years, and neither has Robert and time is short—we have to chance moving her."

"You'll kill her," Mel said. "We all know that. She's already septic. If we don't remove the source of her infection, she'll end up dead."

Robert's mind buzzed with a thousand thoughts, but only one prevailed. All the other surgeries they'd done were for gunshot or stab wounds. They were emergency surgeries, and it was always to locate the bleeder and stabilize the villager before they transferred them out.

But this was different. They were relying on a clinical finding of appendicitis and were going to slice into a young girl with no clear diagnosis.

The alternative, though, could be death.

"Robert knows I got grandfathered into emergency medicine," Mel pushed on. "I did my residency in surgery and switched to the ER. I've done dozens of off-the-cuff appendectomies."

"When? Thirty years ago?" Guillermo shook his head. "Your hands shake like a drunk's. I'm not letting some hospital paper pusher who hasn't seen the inside of an operating room in years cut into this girl."

"I hear you," Mel said. "But I can talk you or Robert through the procedure. It's not brain surgery—it's an appendix."

There was silence as Guillermo fumed and pondered, casting quick glances at the worsening girl. In the silence, Robert realized he agreed with Mel.

"She won't survive the trip," Mel said quietly to Guillermo, "but she might survive the operation."

Just then Maria bellowed a great moan.

"Come on, Guillermo," Mel said, "I know what I'm doing. Let's get on it. Give the poor kid a shot."

"You two do it," Guillermo said. "But if the girl dies, I'll make you both wish you had, too."

And he stormed off.

CHAPTER 13

"First step," Mel said. "Get her sedated. You have fentanyl?"

"Of course." Robert turned to reach into the closet and pull out a vial.

"Excellent," Mel said. "Use just enough so we can do a local and get the surgery going."

Robert pulled off fifty micrograms of the opioid and introduced it into the IV. Fentanyl was just the thing for conscious sedation: quick acting and easy to reverse or adjust, depending on the patient's comfort. And it didn't affect blood pressure as much as opiates such as morphine or Dilaudid.

"Now tell me you know how to do a lidocaine block," Mel said.

"Come on, boss," Robert scoffed. "I'm not a medical student."

"Lidocaine is great when you don't have an anesthesiologist handy. Anesthesiologists like it, too. For women in labor or for doing a C-section."

"Let's get on with it," Robert said.

"Piece of cake," Mel said, his voice reassuring. "It won't put her out, but it'll bury the pain."

Robert probed for her fourth and fifth lumbar vertebrae, covered the area with Betadine, pierced the space between the vertebrae with a syringe and injected the lidocaine.

Quick and effective.

Robert stood and exhaled, revved with the pleasure emergency work always brought him.

"Well done," Mel said. "Now we prep her."

"Let me nurse for you," Yolanda said.

Mel looked inquiringly at Robert, who nodded quickly. Yolanda, a distant cousin of Guillermo's, assisted in most of their medical procedures. Her instincts were as reliable as daylight.

Mel nodded back and set Yolanda up with the prep equipment. She disrobed Maria—who now had a serene but distant gaze—and covered her waist and chest with a sterile sheet. Robert stocked the IV with two grams of the antibiotic Cefepime while Yolanda drenched the girl's abdomen with Betadine. Robert and Mel donned surgical gowns, masks, and gloves. Yolanda closed the tent windows, enclosed the operating arena with mosquito netting, then sat and took Maria's hand.

"Do you remember your landmarks?" Mel's voice was slightly muffled from the surgical mask.

Robert placed one index finger on the thin upper protrusion of the girl's right hipbone—the anterior superior iliac spine—and his other in her umbilicus. He estimated a third of the way between the two fingers. "McBurney's Point."

"A-plus." Mel handed him a syringe. "I placed some epinephrine with the lidocaine—to keep the blood vessels constricted, help keep the lidocaine within the local area. Ice her up good with that. She'll need it."

Maria winced when the needle went into her stomach, but then the fentanyl quickly short-circuited the pain and she went back to semiconsciousness. Robert injected fifteen milliliters of the lidocaine-epinephrine mixture at McBurney's Point and the rest a centimeter deeper.

"Okay, now the fun part." Mel pointed to the area. "Open appendectomy. Three-centimeter incision. No bovie or electrocautery to control the bleeding, so work fast. I'll retract. The way you find the appendix is by …"

"Locating the proximal aspect of the ascending colon. I know."

"But before then you have to …"

"Dissect through the external obliques, blunt dissect, and spread the muscle before hitting the fascia."

Mel raised an eyebrow. "You sure you've never done one of these things before?"

Robert smiled. It was times like this that he was grateful for his photographic memory. He recalled reading the ABCs of an appendectomy on *Schwartz's Principles of Surgery* during his surgery rotation. Typically, most of the surgery attendings were egomaniacs and never let him or the other medical students do anything but retract, so he had to learn the procedure on his own.

With a hand as firm as the blade he held, Robert made the incision. He dissected down to the fascia, which he pierced with blunt scissors. Despite the bleeding, he was able to locate the appendix.

It was three times its normal size, angry and inflamed.

"Surprised it hasn't ruptured," Mel said.

"It's thinking hard about it." Robert deftly isolated it. He was in the zone now, every move streaming from the previous one. He carefully removed the infected appendix and placed it in the bin that Yolanda, with her usual perfect timing, already held out.

"Beautiful work, Roberto," she said.

"Thank you."

She smiled at him over her shoulder as she took the bin outside the netting. Mel peered inside Maria's open abdomen as Robert poured saline into it, then used a sterile syringe to draw as much fluid as he could. Still in the flow, he closed with Vicryl sutures, quickly and with perfect precision.

"Amazing, Robert." Mel clapped him lightly on the back.

"Next forty-eight hours are going to be critical." Robert gazed at Maria's peaceful face. She was sleeping.

"Right," Mel said. "But by getting that bad puppy out and giving her antibiotics, we've nixed most of the sepsis."

"Poor kid." Anger at the traffickers pulled Robert down from his natural high.

"She's lucky we saved her. She would've died without medical care."

Robert shook his head in disgust. "With the narcos, she would've died regardless."

"Let's just pray she doesn't go into total organ failure," Mel said.

"I agree." Robert placed a sterile dressing on the wound.

"You would've made one hell of a surgeon." Mel backed away from the bed, snapped off his gloves and undid his gown.

Robert realized his forehead was dripping with sweat. He wiped his face with his balled up gown and smiled. A feeling spread inside him that he recognized and welcomed—a rock-solid confidence the patient would be okay.

CHAPTER 14

Robert dreamt of skiing down a long, silken slope of peach-colored snow. At the bottom, fast approaching, five trails branched off. He was almost at the intersection when he realized he was skiing down the arm of a giant angel, a smiling creature who enjoyed playing with him. As he reached her wrist she flipped him into the air and he soared chuckling through crystalline snowflakes, then slowly descended and detected the sound of Sharon's laughter.

He landed perfectly in a forest clearing, the snow gone, his skis gone, but Sharon's laugh continued, mixing with jungle sounds. No matter where he looked or how close the sound seemed, he couldn't find her, and he woke suffused in a sadness that clung to him like smoke to the clothes of a firefighter.

He washed his face briskly, trying to shake off the dream. He looked in the metal mirror over the basin and saw a man who didn't have what it took to smile. He dried his face angrily and hurried through the dusk of daybreak to the hospital tent.

Mel sat at Maria's bedside, watching her motionless form. "She okay?" Robert asked anxiously.

"Yes, good. She's good," Mel whispered, not looking away from her.

Robert sat by Mel and they both looked at Maria for a while. "Her breathing has slowed."

"Yolanda just gave her another round of Cefepime," Mel explained. "Meantime, she's got great urine output, even woke up a bit an hour ago and smiled. Showed some energy, perky even. We'll see if she can tolerate fluids in a few hours and go from there."

Robert gently felt the girl's wrist. Her heart rate was down to sixty. "That's a quick turnaround."

"Infection down, health comes round." Mel yawned and stretched. "You get some sleep?"

"A little," Robert said. "I could only get through your wife's charts once before I conked out. The case is trickier than I thought."

"Don't I know it?" Mel shook his head. "It's baffled a whole hospital of doctors for a couple of weeks, so don't feel bad if it takes you more than a few minutes to solve it. I'm grateful for any time you can give it. I know you got a lot going on here but, as you can imagine, I'm eager to get back to her."

"I don't expect it to take much longer," Robert said. "Just a little longer than I thought, that's all."

"Good." It was clear Mel was trying to rustle up some enthusiasm, but he was too tired to feel it.

"Get some sleep, boss," Robert said. "I'm rested. I'll take this shift."

"Thanks," Mel said. "But don't let me sleep too long …"

"Your nap will have to wait."

Guillermo stood in the doorway, backlit by a red sun. He looked like a god of war.

"Are you checking up on us?" Mel smiled. "Look for yourself. The girl is doing great."

Guillermo scowled and stomped in. "Yolanda can watch the girl. You two come with me."

"Come on, Guillermo," Robert pleaded. "Let Mel sleep for a bit."

"I can definitely use it," Mel said.

"It won't take long, Dr. Weiss. Then you can get your beauty sleep."

"Cut the guy some slack, Guillermo," Robert said. "He's been up all night."

"Let's go. *Both* of you." Guillermo wheeled around and left the tent.

"It's okay, Robert." Mel grabbed his sweatshirt and followed Guillermo. "I was a resident once. I can go without sleep."

CHAPTER 15

Guillermo led them northwest of the village, through a trail Robert had forgotten about. Though the jungle was thick with vegetation, Robert had learned it had thousands of secret trails—some made by animals, many more by humans. Some were unkempt, some were as wide and comfortable to walk along as a city street—a partially obstructed maze hewn and hacked by centuries of jungle natives.

Robert was impressed that Mel kept up with Guillermo's warrior pace. He didn't know where or why Guillermo was leading them on this path. But he didn't mind. His heart beat strongly, and the air gave him the light feeling that a heavy drinker looks for but never quite finds in the bottle.

Robert began thinking of his mother. Marching through a grove of sapodilla trees that stood slim and straight as fingers pointed to the heavens, he listened to the rustling of the leaves: they seemed to whisper in his mother's voice that this was sacred ground.

Robert had to blink back tears as an image materialized in his mind's eye.

His mother held his hand while they walked through the little glen behind their house. He heard her melodious voice reciting poetry to him and his little brother.

Our birth is but a sleep and a forgetting.

It was her favorite, a poem by William Wordsworth.

"'Ode: Intimations of Immortality'," Robert muttered.

"What's that?" Mel asked, two steps behind him.

"Nothing, Mel. Just making a mental note. Sorry."

"No problem," Mel said, and they trudged on in silence.

But Robert's head was anything but silent, ringing with his mother's voice weaving Wordsworth's "Ode" around his brain like a cocoon. He was struck with wonder that a mother would speak such a classic English poem so often to her young sons. At the time, of course, it had seemed perfectly natural, as if that was what mothers did. But now it hit him hard how odd it was, and how grateful he was for it.

The poem was her refuge from depression. It made her life worth living.

But Robert's mother and younger brother were brutally murdered by Robert's stepfather, something Robert would never get over.

It was as if she knew her murder was coming and recited that poem line by line to prepare for it.

Robert winced as he walked, remembering the look in her eyes when she recited the lines to him: a mixture of bravery and dread. She always feared her husband, but speaking those lines made the bravery look stronger than the fear. That poem was her antidepressant before the current age of pills. She'd recite it on every walk they took, giving a little explanation after each stanza. Robert liked the explanations. Sometimes he asked questions, despite the tendency of her gaze to drift into the distance, which made it seem she were talking more to herself than to him.

Consoling herself for the beatings, the rape, the abuse.

And now he saw her halt, plop on the ground, and gently pull him down beside her, chanting:

Though nothing can bring back the hour
of splendor in the grass, of glory in the flower;
We will grieve not, rather find
strength in what remains behind.

"Remember those words." Then she repeated them again. "Nature always feels sympathy for you when life gets hard. I love you—and so does nature and you must think of me when you are in nature, teaching you when you want to know something, making you feel better when you're sad. When you think of me, don't think of me as sad, think of me as nature and never forget that 'even the meanest flower that blows can give thoughts that often lie too deep for tears.'"

Robert began to take deeper and deeper breaths as he walked, remembering her with the taste of the rich, dawn-fresh air. He looked around and appreciated the many shades of green now lit by the rising sun, the stripes of light that slanted through the trees, the many birds and crickets and frogs that sang hello to the new day. His heart lifted in his chest. His mother was right. She had given him a timeless gift, a lifeline to nature that so many times had towed him away from despair.

He closed his eyes and took a last deep breath, feeling a spreading calm.

And opened them just in time to avoid walking into Guillermo, who had stopped abruptly.

Mel walked up to them and stopped as well.

The three of them stood there silently, on the crest of a hill, looking down.

"What is this place?" Mel asked. "It makes me want to kneel."

"*El Campo de los Muertos*," Guillermo said.

Mel gave Robert a questioning look.

"The Field of the Dead," Robert said.

CHAPTER 16

They had climbed to a precipice overlooking the jungle and a field dense with trees and crosses made of sticks stuck in the ground. Robert remembered coming there twenty years ago, when he first arrived in Guatemala, toward the end of its atrocious civil war. The trees had been much smaller then and looked more vulnerable. Now they towered over the crosses like watchful, immoveable guardians.

"They came at night." Guillermo stared at the horizon. The morning sun splashed the sky with purples and reds. "Thirty of them. Maybe more. Big, unshaven older guys and a whole lot of kids barely growing hair on their faces. High on something, really excited about their guns, waving machetes around. All wearing camouflage. Screaming and commanding, spit flying out of their mouths, kicking doors down, shooting and hacking at everyone they found—except the women they wanted to rape first. At any given moment it seemed a third of them had their pants down, and a third were zipping up."

Robert looked forlornly in the distance, where a slice of ocean sparkled a bit from the sun, as if just waking up. He remembered when Guillermo had first told him the story of this place. It was after they defended their village against marauders posing as guerillas. Robert had refused to kill their leader, who had cut the right arm off one of the village boys. Robert had chosen to shoot him in the kneecap instead. Guillermo shot the man dead and then yelled at Robert, who had argued that coldly killing another human being was wrong. At the time, Robert believed this.

But that would soon change.

"I was seven." Guillermo turned to face Mel full on. "One guy pulled my hair and turned my head so I could see my father getting shot in the face. I screamed and tried to look away, but he just pulled my hair tighter and yanked my head around so I could see another guy raping my mother while another burned her with a lit cigar. I pulled away and left a hunk of my hair in the guy's hand and ran to save her but then something slammed my head and I went out.

"When I came to, my whole family was dead. I got up, dizzy but still able to walk. The whole village was as gory and awful as they had left our hut. Naked, bloody corpses and body parts all over the place. My aunts and uncles, my childhood friends, neighbors, the good ones and the ones I didn't like—all dead. Slaughtered. The bastards didn't have any mercy. They raped everyone they wanted, seeded our ground with corpses, then looted the place top to bottom. Who was missing? I kept wondering. They didn't get everyone, did they? I worked it out, figured out who wasn't among the dead. Can you guess? It was all the older kids. You know, older but still young. I couldn't figure why. Did they escape? Were they going to come back and save me? I never found them and they never came, and we know why. They were kidnapped and sold, probably as sex slaves." Guillermo's jaw clenched and he locked eyes with Mel.

They stared at each other, neither turning away, until tears made rivulets down Mel's cheeks.

"A jaguar comes into our village," Guillermo said softly, "and begins mauling children, we kill it. Rabid humans should get the same treatment. You might say my childhood trauma dehumanized me, but it's the opposite. It opened my eyes to the reality, which is that there are murdering psychopaths and they come in packs. They need to be put down. Sane men are men of action. What's insane and dehumanizing is apathy. Apathy lets ravenous animals run the earth. Only action keeps good men in charge.

"Too many people just watch bad things happen and don't do anything about it because they're lazy, they don't want to be bothered, they don't think it affects them. They don't think about the big picture. They're animals, too. They're sloths. I'm not—and neither is Robert. Whether you like it or not, Dr. Weiss, the real facts are indisputable. Last night Robert and I saved hundreds of girls from being raped and tortured and driven to despair and insanity. *Hundreds!* We also saved their families and friends from the despair that sets in when your loved ones are tortured and sold as sex toys. I don't regret one single thing about last night—and neither does Robert."

Mel turned to Robert, who nodded calmly.

The sun had risen over the tallest trees. The beauty was a stark contrast to Guillermo's story. Robert's heart ached. Hearing the story again brought home why he felt so attached to his teacher. Each had seen his mother beaten and raped and murdered in cold blood.

"I spent my childhood being passed from tribe to tribe." Guillermo's fearless voice rang through the forest. "Each one terrified of the wild animals around that had forfeited their humanity. I saw all the dying and the wounded and started learning medicine. I made myself remember every detail of every attack on our villages and did all I could to learn the art of war. By the time I was sixteen, I had stopped all attacks on our villages. And I've continued to do that all these years. But I don't know how much longer I can keep it up. Some big cancer is eating this jungle. Too many traffickers high on drugs, little minds with huge weapons who think people are grapes to be stomped for wine to get drunk on."

Guillermo turned from Mel and stared at the distance without saying anything further.

"You're right," Mel finally offered. "There are people who … when we look back at the things they did, we pray to God we could go back in time and bury them alive. I get it. My grandparents were Holocaust survivors. Every story they told me about what was done to them and others, what they lived through, changed my blood somehow, hooked me right up to some kind of rage IV. Never again! That's what you're saying. I get it."

Robert clapped Mel on the shoulder and nodded.

When will it end? How long will evil keep infesting us, calling us to greater work and courage?

Guillermo pivoted and looked past Mel. He took a knife from somewhere inside his pant leg.

Robert followed Guillermo's gaze. "Someone's coming." He took two steps forward and studied the horizon, pulling up his own knife. At the same time he tried to work out his exit strategy. There were only three of them, two who could fight. Mel was dead weight, so they would have to face their attackers square on.

He stood on high alert, listening to a quiet rustling heading their way. Then he let out a huge sigh of relief at the same time Guillermo spoke.

"It's Armando."

A few seconds later Armando appeared and hurried up to his father and whispered something.

"What's going on?" Robert asked.

"Tell them," Guillermo said to his son.

"Another group of traffickers. This one bigger."

"Mel," Robert said, "go back with Armando and get some sleep. Guillermo and I have a little errand to run."

This time Mel didn't object.

CHAPTER 17

"All adults," Robert said, looking through his binoculars at the group trekking through the forest below. "No kids this time."

"No hostages?" Guillermo whispered.

"Seems that way." Robert handed the binoculars over. "It's odd."

Guillermo peered at the men two hundred yards away. "Five guards in front, five in back, all in camouflage, all packing," Guillermo said. "Who are those seven in the middle?"

"Look more like tourists, right?"

"Cargo pants, hiking boots—yeah. Lugging heavy bags."

"Must be equipment of some sort," Robert said.

"Drugs or weapons."

"I'm not sure." Robert took back the binoculars. He jacked up the magnification and looked again. "Something about the bulges in those sacks makes me think equipment. Either way …"

"I know." Guillermo studied the terrain below. "The middle guys are innocent until proven filthy."

Robert shook his head, smiling despite himself. They would kill the armed guards first. That would reveal if the middle seven were good or bad. If they reached for guns from their sacks, he and Guillermo would pick them off with a shower of arrows.

"Let's get closer," Guillermo said. "Hike up higher and take them out as they cross the stream." He led the way up the hill, trekking parallel to the men below.

After a minute of climbing, they reached a precipice overlooking the valley below.

"This is perfect," Robert whispered. "Packed with trees, they can't see us. We can see them. They won't know what hit them."

Guillermo crouched in front of him, carefully shoving aside foliage to make a space to aim through.

Robert propped himself against a massive trunk to help stabilize his grip on the bow. He deftly leaned a dozen arrows upright at his side.

Twelve bulls-eyes a minute.

He knew his rate.

This won't take long.

He steadied his breathing.

He notched an arrow, pulled it back, and stuck the tip through the leaves, sighting the chest of the first guard.

What just happened?

There were now only two guards in front and two in back.

Then came a quick rustling and a muffled yelp nearby. Robert felt a cold, hard ring of steel on his right temple.

"Slacken the arrow, Dr. McKenzie, or I'll spray those leaves with your brains."

CHAPTER 18

The barrel dug into Robert's temple. Out of the corner of his eye, Robert detected a short man in a camouflage hoodie at the other end of the AK-47, backed by more men holding Guillermo at gunpoint.

"So you're the gringo doctor messing everything up for us," Shorty said.

Robert slowly released the string of his bow. "So you're the bastard who's been raping and torturing children."

The thug jerked his rifle back and slammed the butt hard into Robert's temple.

Robert collapsed, a pulsing migraine erupting in a flash. His vision blurred. The flaring pain made him want to claw his head open to let it out. He gritted his teeth with the effort and lifted his hand to check for a head wound, but Shorty stomped the hand with his boot. "Keep your hands where I can see them, Dr. McKenzie." He looked at Guillermo. "Dr. Martinez, you've recruited another sucker, I see. Did you give him the same candy-ass shit you used to force-feed me and my brothers years ago?"

Robert's vision started clearing, and he saw Guillermo's eyes narrow into dangerous slits. "Rimaldi?"

The man brought down his hood. He had a pasty face, beady eyes and a small, pink nose.

"I'm surprised you remember me, old man. I was no more your favorite than you were mine. You know you always had a bad smell, like bleach?"

"Anything clean stinks to someone with the nose of a rat."

"Ironic, isn't it, that your favorite pupil was my little brother Manny—the one you killed yesterday?"

Robert painfully sat up. "Guillermo," he rasped, swaying a bit. "This guy, he's … he's …?"

"Please, Dr. Bleach," Rimaldi said. "Care to catch your latest student up on the success of your after-school program? About what a great man your teaching formed in me?"

Guillermo spat.

Rimaldi stepped forward and slapped him.

"Respect, old man. Respect. That's what you always taught us."

"I can't respect anyone who enjoys hitting old men held at gunpoint."

Rimaldi took a slow deep breath, glaring at Guillermo. "No use talking to you. My words can't get past all the hair in your ears." He turned his narrowed eyes to Robert and spoke with a voice just a pinch below a whine. "I tried, Dr. McKenzie. I wanted to learn. The jungle was killing us. I wanted to learn about machetes and guns, but he just kept talking about leaves and flowers and seeds. My stupid brothers and I were close family friends with him and his ex-wife, that *puta* Rivera, who spoke a retarded kind of Spanish. You shipped her out of here, didn't you, Guillermo? Said you were afraid some enemy would go after her, but really it was because she kind of smelled, right? Like a pig? Just like you do now. Guilt sweat because you killed your student, my brother, and now I'm going to kill your student and then roast you to death over a slow fire."

"You're an interesting guy, Rimaldi," Robert said, "Before you kill me, though, would you give me something to go out with? No harm. I mean your philosophy. How can you possibly justify what you do?"

Rimaldi looked at Robert with a combination of arrogance and amusement, his eyes jumpy and energized. "We're making a lot of money and doing some good." His speech sounded pressured, likely from methamphetamine. "Simply said, I have a brilliant business partner. Brilliant because he's a realist. He follows the law of the jungle. You guys have no idea how much you've cost our operation, not just financially. You've clogged our fucking arteries. You've wasted a lot of the time we need for this project, which has worldwide importance."

"Smuggling drugs and trafficking girls?" Guillermo scoffed. "I should've known you were a loser the day I caught you twisting that gecko's head off."

"I was learning medicine, which is more than you ever taught me." Rimaldi laughed. "There is still so much for us to do. Beyond even all my money, women, drugs, and a mansion in Guatemala City. Very soon we're going to be celebrities. Famous. We might win a Nobel Prize for our project."

"A Nobel Prize?" Robert faked a look of awe that he could see pleased Rimaldi and stole side glances at Guillermo. They had a sign protocol. Guillermo's subtle hand gestures signaled a particular divide and conquer procedure.

To begin in less than a minute.

"You know why you talk loud, Rimaldi?" Guillermo asked. "Because there's this whisper in your ear you can't stand." Guillermo shut his eyes tightly for a moment. "It's telling you you're going to hell."

Saw it, Guillermo. Thirty seconds and counting.

"There's no whisper!" Rimaldi shouted.

The men agreed automatically with grunts and answers of no.

"They're a bunch of ass-kissers," Guillermo went on, wiping his right eyebrow with an index finger.

I take Rimaldi, he takes the men.

"They don't like you any more than we do," Guillermo said. "It's how cartels work. Any one of these guys will take you out the first chance they get. You're crazy if you think any of these men has any loyalty."

"You're a fool, old man. My partner and I are going to run this jungle. And people are going to love us for it. We've already taken over the drug trade and now it's on to bigger and better."

"Human trafficking?" Robert rasped, acting puzzled, jiggling his legs, getting ready. "Is that really bigger and better? Being a slave trader? Isn't that, I don't know, like so 1700s?"

"If that's all you think we're up to, you're dumber than that old goat." Rimaldi brayed, pointing his gun at Guillermo. "The one who taught me will be indirectly responsible for creating an empire and destroying this jungle. Take *that* to your grave."

"Even your parents couldn't stand you, Rimaldi. They'd come to me, wanting to throw you down the well, smother you in your bed, poison your rice and beans. Can you blame them? Your mother used to say you were a miscarriage that didn't die."

"She never said that!" Rimaldi rushed at Guillermo, waving his gun.

The two guards flanking Guillermo scurried out of the way.

Action!

With one swift move, Robert levered to his knees, pulled the knife from behind his neck, and threw it between Rimaldi's second and third vertebrae, causing instant paralysis.

As Rimaldi collapsed, Guillermo grabbed his body, twisted it around, and pointed the AK-47 at the remaining five men, showering them with bullets.

Ten seconds later, all six bloody carcasses carpeted the ground.

CHAPTER 19

Robert heard distant yelling and commotion.

The others!

There was rapid gunfire. Bullets sliced through branches and leaves, ricocheting off rocks.

The two men dropped to the ground simultaneously. Guillermo pulled himself to Robert's side. Only a few bullets were close.

Always difficult to aim accurately uphill.

"How many left?" Guillermo asked.

More bullets sprayed in a wide range around them. One tore through Rimaldi's dead face.

"Four men with those." Robert indicated the AK-47 Guillermo had wrested from Rimaldi's clutches. "And the seven civilians."

The shots came less frequently, striking farther from where they lay.

Then silence.

Then almost inaudible murmurs and swooshes, fading.

"We can't let them escape!" Robert jumped to his feet. Being so close to death had renewed his sense of purpose and released a ton of adrenaline, which doused his head pain. He snatched his bow and quiver as Guillermo struggled upright.

"Meet you down there," Robert yelled, running off.

His legs were strong and his body felt light. He fancied himself a predator—a great lion bounding down the hill, eyeing a flock of elands scattering below.

Lions had claws and teeth.

He had arrows.

One of the armed men heard him thrashing down the hill, turned, and lifted his barrel.

Before the barrel rose to waist level, Robert had reached into his quiver and positioned the bow. He let go two arrows in rapid succession. One arrow pierced the man's solar plexus, the second bore through his left eye.

One down, three to go.

Robert didn't slacken his speed on the forested incline for a second, but his enemies had too much of a head start. He could barely make out their retreating backs disappearing over a faraway crest.

Too far to shoot, too many trees between us.

They're only scrambling. I could be flying.

He wrapped the bow over his shoulder and sprinted to the next overhang. He leapt off, soaring down to the lowlands, both hands free and outstretched. As slender branches and thick leaves slapped at his face, he had a choice of three wrist-thick vines to grab. He had done this for fun in his early years studying with Guillermo. His mentor had frowned on the practice, but Robert couldn't resist testing his gymnastic skills on the vines, even yahooing from time to time at the tree creatures that clambered away.

A split second before he reached the vines, he saw that there was one on his left that hung free and longest, and he gripped it firmly with both hands, his bow thumping comfortably into his back at the slight deceleration. The vine lurched forward with his momentum, and he arched his back and kicked out, giving it extra thrust.

Seconds later he let go and sailed toward the next opportune vine, already swinging forward with two howler monkeys clinging to it. They chittered nervously at his approach and jumped aside as he latched on a few feet above where they had been. This vine was green and slightly slippery, and he slid three yards before getting a handhold, twirling some, losing his orientation for a few moments.

When he finally stopped spinning, he caught a glimpse of a camouflage flak suit hacking through thick foliage a hundred yards ahead.

With a great oomph, he kicked and whipped again, and the vine catapulted him into space. He quickly notched an arrow and let it fly as he flew toward an intricate array of vines, then tucked his bow once more behind him. He heard a blood-draining yelp ahead but didn't dare look. He had to concentrate. His gaze remained on his chosen vine, which he neared at blur speed.

Reach. Grab. Clasp.

Robert swung over a dizzying ravine lined with shards of shale that looked like shark teeth coming up to devour him. As he rose from the nadir of the swing, he saw the guard stagger with an arrow in his neck, try to pull it out, then pitch headlong down into the ravine.

Up ahead, two o'clock.

Another vine waited for him as poised as the next teammate in a relay race. Robert snap-kicked and launched toward it, scanning the area for more guards as he glided, spotting one. Midair, Robert pulled out an arrow with one hand. He snatched the rough-barked vine with the other, wrapping the supple vine around his bow-arm as he swung with it: notching, flexing, aiming, shooting, hitting the man in the upper left back, piercing his heart, forcing him to the ground. Seeing the man struggle to stand, Robert slid down to the bottom of the vine and dropped ten angling feet to land a perfect flying kick to the man's chest, arresting for good any feeble cardiac function he had left. Robert's momentum tumbled him forward, but after a couple of somersaults he came to a controlled landing in a patch of ferns.

Three down, one to go.

Robert jabbed the knuckles of his right hand into the ground, swiveled, got his feet under him and took off in a full sprint in the direction of the last narcotraficante. He weaved through small gaps in the big trunks, splashed through a stream alive with snakes that slithered away from his ruckus, and huffed and puffed up a slope buzzing with wasps the size of his little finger. There he surprised a gaudy gang of macaws flapping madly into the bright sunlight and stopped dead as a racket of automatic fire stitched the ground five yards ahead of him. He dove behind a tree just as more fire pockmarked its trunk.

He crouched low, his back at the base of the tree, letting himself calm. A half mile behind him he saw a moving dot.

Guillermo!

The dot's movement was fluid, hitchless, sure-footed.

Like water seeking the valley.

Even in his seventies, Guillermo still moved like an Olympic decathlete, with the same Zen alacrity he had instilled in Robert years ago.

The shooting had stopped. Robert peered around the tree, bow and arrow at ready. He glimpsed a camouflage pant leg, moving away.

Too far to fire.

He noticed the other men, the ones not in camouflage with the hiking gear. They were scampering ahead of the armed guard, who was now in full relief against a patch of sky. Robert didn't want to chance a shot because he wasn't sure about the unarmed men. They were running scared as if they had no experience with gunfire or combat. Robert couldn't shake the impression that they were civilians.

Were they teamed with the traffickers or their hostages?

Robert lit out from behind the tree and began pursuing the strange group, watching the armed guard turn from time to time to fire blindly in Robert's direction. It made Robert cautious but not afraid. The bullets came nowhere near him, and he always had plenty of time to hide behind a rock or tree when he saw the guard turn.

It soon became clear the guard was shepherding the hostages toward the Mayan ruins at Kundal, prodding them past warning signs and site barriers.

What were civilians doing in the jungles of Guatemala?

Another spray of gunfire cut into a grove not ten yards from him. When Robert peered ahead again, he saw the whole group now running. He tore from behind his protective boulder and sped ahead. He was determined to find out what this group was up to. He couldn't help but wonder if it was connected to the "empire" that rat-faced Rimaldi had blabbered about.

Robert's adrenaline had drained somewhat with all the stopping and starting, and his head throbbed powerfully where Rimaldi had butted him. He forced himself to speed up. He was only four hundred yards behind and saw that the last shooter was prodding the civilians to run faster.

That made Robert break into a sprint.

But he wasn't gaining on the escapees any more.

To his right was another cliff edge, a sturdy tree just ten yards off it with a branch over which dangled a fat vine. It beckoned him. Without another thought he ran full tilt toward it and jumped. For a breathless moment it was as if time had stopped and all that remained was the wind in his face and the dead silence of the yawning chasm beneath. Then he came down on the thick branch, slipped but grabbed the vine and pulled himself upright. He backed up to the trunk then ran to the end of the branch and swung toward another tree, under which the escaping group had passed seconds ago.

His feet landed on the far end of it, and the branch bent with his weight, but he felt balanced enough to let go of the vine and reach for the next one.

But then there was a cracking sound.

Not of gunfire, but of wood.

Before he could grab the neighboring vine, Robert sensed himself falling.

His adrenalized perception numbed all pain. A slow-motion parade of options went through his mind.

Branches, leaves, sharp pokes. Whatever he grabbed whisked out of his hands.

Small branch, tangled vine, leaves.

Thirty feet in free fall.

Then twenty.

Stinging slaps, light brushes, brutal jolts, myriad branches, loud thrashing, and soft sounds of windfall.

Ten.

Loud sounds of cracking branches.

Five.

Jabbing pain, sudden fear.

One.

Solid earth.

Blackout.

CHAPTER 20

"Come on, Tarzan. Get up!"

Robert felt a kick at his feet. His body was a torn sack of pain and his head threatened to explode.

"How many times have I told you those branches are for little monkeys, not big apes," Guillermo went on. "Monkeys are smaller and lighter and a hell of a lot more agile than you." He shook his head and sighed heavily. "Hello? Earth to Tarzan?"

Robert opened his eyes. Light shot into his brain like Lilliputian arrows. The world looked hazy. The green forest suddenly began seesawing and he felt seasick. Guillermo put a canteen to his lips. The water tasted wonderful, but the trees above him looked like they were bending down to grab him, their branches groping monstrously at him. He felt nauseated and dizzy.

He took another gulp and started to feel the tiniest bit less than awful.

His doctor persona kicked in, as if he were an internist waking up from a catnap at the end of a twenty-four–hour shift. Still hazy, he began to assess any damage.

Positive loss of consciousness.

Do I have an intracranial bleed? Epidural or subdural hematoma? A skull fracture?

He lifted an arm to feel for any indentation in his head and didn't note any. He felt the back of his neck: no midline tenderness. He had sensation in all four limbs.

They're all throbbing, but is there a fracture?

He tested their movement and noted he had normal motor function as long as he didn't mind the urge to scream. Nonetheless, no bones stuck out, so there were no distracting injuries. He reassessed his cervical spine, slowly lifting his hand toward the back of his neck and palpating each cervical vertebra separately.

"Enough, Roberto. Get up. I've already assessed you. You don't have a spinal fracture, an intracranial bleed, or any intra-abdominal pathology. There are no extremity fractures. Come on, let's go."

Robert patted the ground beneath him—thick, lush carpet of high jungle grass. He looked up. Many of the thick lower branches had snapped and bent as they slowed his fall. He sat up slowly, rolling his neck around. He felt stinging needles shooting from his lower brain down through his spine.

Head pain suddenly took over.

The rifle slam plus the fall.

He put his head between his knees until the searing bolt in his cerebellum dimmed. Gently, he placed a hand over his scalp and began massaging it while assessing for lacerations, hematomas, and step-offs.

"You already checked for intracranial bleed," Guillermo said. "And I've checked for that and everything else. Trust my clinical assessment and get your ass up."

"Your compassion moves me greatly."

"Come on. We're done here. Those bastards are too far away. Let's head back to the village."

Robert forced himself up. The number of aches in his body was astonishing, made even worse by the fact that each time he got hurt this badly, all the ghosts of his previous injuries seemed to rise up and join in all the fun. The kidney bruisings from his abusive stepfather; the wounds and blows the guerillas gave him during the Guatemalan Civil War; the damages he earned in his years fighting crime in Manhattan.

"Sorry, Guillermo. Those guys escaped because of me. One guard and those seven others."

"It's all right," Guillermo said, without a trace of enthusiasm.

They began walking. Robert limped at first, but corrected his gait before long so Guillermo wouldn't harass him. After trudging a few minutes in silence, Robert spoke. "So that Rimaldi. Lost cause? What was his story?"

"Brother of the one I killed yesterday." A tortured sadness suffused Guillermo's face. "Little Manny and Rimi. My best friend's sons. Lost cause indeed."

"You teach what you can, right? The rest is up to them."

"Rimaldi. *Bad Boy Rimi*, we called him. Middle brother of the trio. Little sadist. Always beating on Manny, kicking dogs. Hated life for some reason. Always talking louder, acting superior. Condescending. Too eager to shout, never willing to listen. The kid had his moments, though. He loved martial arts, got real attentive and humble when we worked with weapons. I thought I could get him to see how that attitude led to better things, but I guess it never took."

"What about the oldest kid?" Robert asked. "What's his name?"

"Joaquin."

"Are we going to run into him, too?"

"That won't happen," Guillermo said fiercely. "Thank God one of them made something of himself. After his father died, Joaquin went to medical school in Guatemala City, then moved to Miami for a surgery residency. Probably finishing up his fellowship now."

"One for three isn't bad."

"In batting, maybe," Guillermo said, "but for life it sucks."

"What about Rimaldi's empire thing? Is that the evil out there you've been sensing?"

"Maybe. I can't say for sure. Bad things are brewing, I know. The narcotraficantes are trying to take over here. Kick out the locals."

"Why?"

"All I can think of is that the jungle makes a perfect cover for their cartel and their trafficking. It would take ten armies to police this place, and even then there would be plenty of places to hide. But I don't know. There must be something else, but I just can't see it. I wish we could've made one of those guys talk. Find out who's behind this blitzkrieg."

"I blew it. Sorry, Guillermo."

"What's done is done."

Robert nodded. They were halfway home now and he was starting to feel semi-human again. "Rimaldi called me by name. How did he know about me?"

"We've been busting their balls for a few weeks. Drug pimps really love their balls. Anybody mess with them, they make it a point of pride to find out who's responsible. You should know that you probably have a hefty prize on your head."

Robert laughed. "I'm in good company. I'm sure the prize on your head is ten times mine."

A moment later, they both froze.

Robert closed his eyes and let his ears tune to the noise.

A rustling. Not like a bird, a monkey, or any animal.

Silence.

Then the sound again.

Robert crept quietly around the tree to look.

The intruder started to run back through the undergrowth.

Robert took off. He heard the man groan loudly. Soon, Robert was flying over boulders and crashing through brush and saplings. He ignored the head throbbing and body aches. The intruder was in sight now. Robert bounded high over a deadfall tree and tackled the gasping man. As their bodies hit the ground, Robert already had his knife at the guy's throat.

"Please don't hurt me!" the man yelled.

It was an American civilian, and he looked petrified.

CHAPTER 21

"Don't kill me!" His voice, with its slight Texas twang, quivered. Tears welled in his eyes and his slender body shook. "I have a family. Wife, two daughters. Pull that knife away. What have I done? Please, don't hurt me!"

Robert didn't move. The blade of his knife pressed into the man's throat as far as it could without piercing the skin. Something was off about this guy, but he didn't know what. He seemed like anything but a drug dealer.

"Who the hell are you?"

"I'm a physician."

"What?" Robert gaped at the man.

"I came out here … to do good."

"Don't move." Robert held the blade right where it was. "And stop squirming or you'll lose your larynx. What kind of physician are you?"

Robert's head spun. He felt confused, a feeling he hated more than anything. Not having a grasp on a situation made him determined to solve it. The uncertainty inherent in emergency medicine drove him to learn more. That's why he studied so hard. Why he spent every waking moment poring over textbooks and medical journals and clinical studies.

The Texan's eyes skittered. The fear he gave off was not just the fear of getting his throat cut.

"Are you going to talk or what?" Robert dug the blade deeper into the man's flesh without breaking the skin.

"Okay, okay … my name is Verne Fox," the man whimpered. "From Austin, Texas. I'm a hepatologist. That's a …"

"Liver specialist," Robert spat out. "I know what a hepatologist is, you dumb motherfucker!"

"Okay," Fox sputtered, looking puzzled. "I'm s-s-sorry. Most people don't."

This guy doesn't know I'm a doctor.

"Talk!" Robert shouted. "What are you doing here? I'll give you ten seconds before I slit your throat."

"It's like … Doctors Without Borders … this nonprofit group I joined, called Giving More. Provides free medical care to remote villages in Central America. Nicaragua last year, this year Guatemala … huge alcoholism problem here, a lot of liver disease, so here I am."

"All those others you were with … are they all hepatologists?"

"No, just me. Others were, let me think … a cardiovascular surgeon, an ophthalmologist, an anesthesiologist, a general surgeon, a pulmonologist … and a nephrologist." Fox was breathing fast, his words coming out in wheezy puffs. "We usually bring nurses, physician assistants, and dental hygienists with us, but only physicians were invited on this trip."

"Why are you all in *this* jungle?"

"I don't know … they brought us here."

Robert's confusion threatened to blind him. He needed to keep his anger in check and stay logical. This guy could have valuable information about the narcotraficantes.

Robert grabbed a hunk of Fox's hair and pulled it tight. "*Who* brought you here? And why?"

"I was picked up at the airport, in Guatemala City. A guy named Rimaldi in a black SUV. The nephrologist and the general surgeon were in it. No one talked. We didn't even look at each other. I thought we were going somewhere in the city, but we kept driving north. I asked where we were going and was told to shut up. We got to Selaute and started hiking. I was hungry and pissed and scared. Then we were met by armed men. They marched us here. Then gunfire, all hell broke loose, we all scattered, you tackled me. And you still have a knife at my throat. If *you* don't know what's going on, I know even less."

"They didn't tell you anything? They abducted you? It's all too hard to believe, Fox."

"It's the truth!"

Nothing the man said lessened Robert's anxiety. What in hell was an American doctor doing in this jungle? Abducted? For what?

He could almost hear Mel and Sharon saying to him in unison: *What are you doing, Robert? Let the poor man breathe.*

Robert let go of his hair, pulled the knife back an inch and stared at the man's eyes. He looked terrified, for sure. But he also looked guilty. And something else was in his eyes, too, something cold and feral, way in the back, watching him in a way that unnerved him.

Something's off.

Is it me or him?

"He's lying." Guillermo had emerged behind him as quietly as a hologram turning solid. "He's one of them. He's not telling the truth. Kill him."

Robert turned around, but kept his knife close to the man's throat.

Is Guillermo playing bad cop to get this guy to talk, or does he mean it?

"I'm not sure, Guillermo. I think he's telling the truth."

"Half-truths are no-truths!" Guillermo came up to Robert's side and pointed at the off-putting man. "He's lying.

Don't let the fact that he looks like your twin dissuade you from ending his life."

With a jolt Robert realized it was true. The guy's build matched Robert's and his face, though beardless, looked roughly the same.

Do I mistrust the guy because he reminds me of myself?

"Come on, Robert!" Guillermo's voice cut through Robert's thoughts like a machete through jungle vines. "This joker is holding something back." He slammed his elbow into the side of Fox's head. "Don't give me that look! You're not fooling me." He rammed his elbow into Fox's other temple.

"Jesus, Guillermo. Take it easy."

"Please," Fox implored. "I told you all I know. I'm a physician. I'm not a terrorist. I don't own a gun. I have a family. I'm as much in the dark about all this as you."

"Robert, are you going to cut his throat or should I?"

"You're serious about killing him?" Robert asked, bewildered. "What if he's telling the truth? And if he isn't, then killing him won't get anything out of him."

"He's not going to talk. I'm a hundred percent sure. He's on lockdown in there. He's shitting in his pants because of someone else, not us. Kill the guy, and let's go home."

"Kill an unarmed guy in cold blood? I'll kill drug lords and sex traffickers, but pardon me if I hesitate to kill an American physician who might be here on a medical mission and who might have information we can use."

"Medical mission?" Guillermo snorted. "That's bullshit. He's not a physician."

Robert stared at Fox. "Name all the anastomosis between the celiac artery and the superior mesenteric artery."

The man gaped at Robert. "What?"

"He's a fake!" Guillermo said. "I told you."

Robert shrugged his shoulders and grabbed Fox's hair again.

"The celiac trunk connects with the common hepatic artery to the gastroduodenal artery." Fox babbled, gazing upward as if he recited from a book in the sky. "Which can anastomose to either the anterior or posterior superior pancreaticoduodenal artery to the pancreas and duodenum. From there the anterior and posterior inferior pancreaticoduodenal artery anastomoses to the inferior pancreaticoduodenal artery and onto the SMA."

In Robert's photographic memory *Netter's Anatomy* opened to the drawing of the abdominal arteries.

"He's right." He let go of the guy's hair.

"Excuse me for taking a few seconds to recall all that," Fox said, "but I'm not used to having a knife at my throat. At the hospital, I usually get questions from a resident or medical student, and my life doesn't depend on the answers."

"Yeah, but someone else's might," Guillermo barked, then went into what looked like a trance.

Robert understood. It was Guillermo's version of the infuriating confusion Robert felt. Things in the jungle were getting more and more bizarre.

First an increase in criminal activity.

More gunmen, expanding drug cartels, a huge spike in sexual trafficking.

Now physicians kidnapped and brought to the jungle.

What exactly is happening?

Guillermo's eyes suddenly cleared and he laid into Robert. "His medical knowledge means he's a doctor. It doesn't mean he's a good one—and he's not here to do good, that's for damn sure. You know and I know he stinks of lies and guilt. He's in league with murderers until proven otherwise. I'm in charge here, and I'm telling you to kill him."

"I can't do it, Guillermo."

"Okay, I'll do it."

Robert pulled away from the man and squared off with Guillermo. "I can't let you do that. He's one of us. He's a physician. Let's just bring him to camp, put him in our prison, and interrogate him. To kill him in cold blood without having all the details ... it's not smart, not good, and not right."

"Don't give me that shit, Robert. Fact is your former boss blunted your edge and that social worker made you all tender."

"She has nothing to do with this."

"She has *everything* to do with it," Guillermo countered. "When you got back from New York, I could tell you'd changed. Your body is here but your mind is there. And your mind wishes your body were there. You practically drooled at the chance to hop on a plane back to Manhattan. You're as half here as Fox is half-telling the truth. You've back-burnered my jungle, so you don't belong here. You should go back with Weiss. I can't work with someone who doesn't obey orders."

"Guillermo, I can't kill a family guy just because you have a hunch."

"One of my hunches was you, when I first met you. How'd that turn out?"

"It led to this."

"Yeah. Bad hunch. You're right. The guy's yours then. Do whatever you want with him."

"Fine," Robert said. "I take full responsibility."

"He takes responsibility," Guillermo mocked and spat. "Okay, then. Here's the deal. When you and your buddy get back to camp, I expect you to pack your things and leave. I want you, this prisoner, and your fat friend out of my village by tomorrow afternoon."

Guillermo walked away, but his voice lingered in the air like poisonous gas.

CHAPTER 22

The village prison was a square hut built of thick logs tightly strapped together, with plate-size windows and a padlocked door. A slender but sturdy tree grew in the middle of the inside area up through a small opening in the corrugated metal roof. Robert tied Fox's hands behind his back and shackled his legs to a chain embedded in the trunk. In the march to the village, Fox had tried to engage Robert in conversation, chatting about the forest and asking Robert how he knew so much about medicine.

Robert had said nothing.

Although he didn't want to kill Fox as Guillermo had ordered, he shared his mentor's unease about the detainee. In the prison hut, Fox had turned belligerent, yelling at his unfair treatment, insisting he was a man of medicine, engaged in the healing arts, calling Robert and Guillermo savages and inhumane for their treatment of him.

Still Robert said nothing. But as he walked out the door, with Fox pleading to have his limbs freed, Robert suddenly turned and fixed him with a stare that shut him up. "You're going to talk, Dr. Fox. You're going to tell us who you fear more than us. Or you're going to waste away here until you do. At some point soon, wasting away will seem worse than being wasted by whatever bogeyman you serve. I'll talk to you when you're a lot hungrier than you are now."

Robert opened the door to leave and Fox started screaming insults, which stopped as soon as Robert turned again. "Stop screaming or we'll tape your mouth shut. Got it?"

Fox glared at him, breathing audibly.

"Got it?" Robert said.

Fox sat there panting, glaring, then said, "You're a sadist."

Robert strode back to Fox, who cringed and flinched.

"Did you just insult me?" Robert asked. "You hang with murderers and human traffickers and carry medical equipment for them and won't tell me why, and you insult me?" Robert slapped Fox hard across the face. "You sit there knowing full well what we need to know to stop terrorists around here and you think you can pass moral judgment?" He slapped him again, and then once more, a hard one-two that cracked like rifle shots through the air. Fox blinked hysterically, speechless with fright. Robert put his face two inches from Fox's, his furious gaze lasering into Fox's brain. "You're guilty of something. I know it, and you know it."

Fox shut his eyes tight, as if waiting for another slap. When it didn't come, he opened them again to evaluate Robert's menace. Robert's hand was no longer raised, and he had backed off. Fox gulped. "I don't know that I am, but I'm sorry for calling you a sadist, even though you seem to think it's fine to slap a man whose hands are tied."

Robert immediately went to a shelf and pulled down a roll of duct tape.

"No, please don't. I'm sorry," Fox whimpered. "Please . . ."

Robert slapped a strip of tape over Fox's mouth and left the hut. Fox's desperate, muffled protests followed him.

Robert locked the door and told the boy manning the prison to rip Fox's tape off in two hours and give him a cup of water. The kid nodded gravely and began tossing the makeshift *fútbol* he always had with him.

A commotion on the other side of the village drew Robert to investigate. There were Mel and Armando, surrounded by a band of raucous village kids. Armando was instructing Mel on how to use the bow and arrow. Mel held the bow awkwardly with one hand, fumbling to fit the beveled end of an arrow into the bowstring.

Robert squeezed through the circle and clapped Mel on his shoulder. "I see you've been entertaining yourself this morning."

"I feel like I'm a kid at summer camp," Mel said, a smile on his face. He finally got the arrow notched, carefully turned with his tongue showing at the side of his mouth, and looked at his target, a thick tree trunk ten yards away. He pulled the string back, his arms and hands tremulous, and spoke in a choked voice. "And Robin Hood splits the tree and wins Maid Marian!" He let go of the string.

The arrow fell short of the trunk by five feet. The kids laughed wildly.

"I'm glad you think our home is a summer camp," Guillermo scoffed and walked away.

Robert shook his head. He hadn't even noticed Guillermo arriving at the scene.

"What's wrong with him?" Mel fumbled to notch another arrow. "Look, Robert, you know as well as anyone that I'm eager to get back to Francine, but I don't want to push you. You got a lot going on, and if you tell me that my wife's coma is temporary and that you'll figure out her diagnosis, then I believe you. I'm trying my hardest to keep my shit together here. Have I done anything to offend Guillermo?"

Robert grimaced, still stinging from Guillermo's scathing remarks in the forest. "We had a rough morning out there. A net full of razors is closing around us, but we can't figure out where it's coming from. We even took a prisoner. A doctor, no less. American."

"An American physician?"

Robert nodded.

"What's he doing here?" Mel asked.

"Not sure," Robert said. "He told us he was kidnapped by one of the major narcotraficantes, but something isn't adding up."

"Is there anything I can do to help?" Mel asked.

Robert shook his head. "It's not your problem. You enjoy your last day in the jungle." He pointed at the bow. "Let's see how you handle that thing."

"All right, but don't get jealous of my skills."

Again, Mel's hands shook as he stretched the string back. He pointed the notched but wavering arrow toward the tree and began a soft groan that crescendoed to a straining whine, which the children mocked in chorus. Then with a karate yowl, he released the arrow and sent it wide. It missed the tree trunk and disappeared into the bushes.

The kids exploded with laughter, some of them falling to the ground, clutching their stomachs. Mel pasted a smile on his face, but Robert could tell he was frustrated.

"You know what could make a big difference?" Robert said to him quietly.

"Yeah," Mel said. "I need about ten thousand hours of practice."

"You need to breathe," Robert said. "You're holding your breath when you start to shoot."

"Oh, come on, Robert. I'm breathing. I'm not dead, am I? Nah, it's the same problem I've had since I was a kid. I'm useless. Two left feet. Not much of an athlete. I was always the kid picked last at games. No hand-eye coordination."

"That's ridiculous," Robert said. "You'd never be the doctor you are without exceptional hand-eye control."

"Really?" Mel looked surprised. "Huh. I never thought about that."

"Try again," Robert ordered. "I'll teach you how it's done."

Mel started to string the arrow, but soon his hands started shaking.

Robert smiled. "Relax, boss. Notch that arrow and breathe nice and easy."

With steady hands, Mel did just that.

"Keep breathing now as you pull the string back, as if you're inhaling it back."

Mel pulled the string back smoothly.

"Now hold steady but exhale, and breathe easy a few times. That's it."

The kids were all still and quiet now, showing an innate respect for the moment, a ritual revolving around essential elements in their lives—a weapon and hunting.

"Keep breathing naturally," Robert instructed, his voice in rhythm with the rise and fall of Mel's chest. "Rest your eyes on the target. You'll feel your body start to adjust. Let it. That's it."

The muscles of Mel's face relaxed.

The quality of your life is dependent on the quality of your breath.

"Good," Robert said. "What's happening now is your hands and arms and shoulders are automatically eyeing the target with you. For that, you need plenty of oxygenation. That's it. That's looking good. One more inhalation. Now let the air out slowly … and release the string."

Thwack!

The arrow hit the lower trunk of the tree.

Silence. Gasps from the kids. Then they all started cheering, some of them running up to Mel and hugging him.

Mel's face broke into a giant smile. He looked at Robert, eyes glowing. "Om," he said.

"That's right," Robert said. "Like meditation."

"Meditation in action."

"You got it." Robert shrugged. "Archery's my yoga."

"I want to try it again." Mel reached for another arrow. The kids backed away and grew silent again.

"Keep practicing, amigo, until it becomes as natural to you as eating." Robert laughed and headed for his hut.

"Wait a second! You need to help me do that again."

"Nah. You're fine. What you just learned is all you need now. Just ingrain it. Do it, then do it again. Listen to the kids cheer. That's all the instruction you'll need for now." Robert yawned. "I'll go over your wife's records and have an answer for you in a few hours."

Mel grew sober, took a deep breath, and nodded. "Thanks, Robert."

"You're welcome, boss. Now carry on."

CHAPTER 23

Robert walked into his hut, took off his shoes, and stretched. Though exhausted, he forced himself to sit at his wooden table and pick up Francine's chart. A mouth-watering aroma teased his nostrils, and he turned and saw a plate of fruit and a large tamale filled with avocado, leftover boar, and hot peppers. The grouchy old one-toothed cook loved Robert and always took pains to make sure he ate enough. Robert didn't know how hungry he was until he bit into the tamale, which was still warm and delicious as usual. He poured himself a splash of Mestizo Mezcal, chomped down a few more bites, and took it all back to the table, where he went through Francine's workup while he ate.

After a while he closed the report, took a deep breath, a sip of the mezcal, and grabbed his notebook, turning to a blank page. He felt like he was back at St. Jude's, eating lunch at his desk as he pored over charts.

He took another sip and wrote down "Altered Mental Status."

This was his favorite chief complaint. The first time he'd seen it was as a third-year student in medical school, during his emergency medicine rotation. EMTs wheeled in a fat male patient in his forties, unresponsive but able to breath on his own.

"Altered mental status," his attending had said right away. "Sleuth out the cause, McKenzie."

He was prepared. He'd gotten excited in his studies whenever he came across this diagnosis because there were so many disease processes that could alter consciousness. Searching out the answer had made him feel like a medical detective, and he had armed himself with a great mnemonic checklist for rooting out the cause of altered mental status: *AEIOU TIPS.*

A = alcohol
E = electrolyte problems (low/high sodium or potassium) or encephalopathy (brain disease from a liver issue or high blood pressure)
I = insulin problems (low/high sugar levels from diabetes or injecting too much insulin)
O = opiates (heroin, Percocet, etc.) or other drugs
U = uremia (high blood urea nitrogen from kidney failure)
T = trauma, temperature (either hypo- or hyperthermia), tumors, thyroid disease
I = infection (encephalitis, sepsis)
P = psychogenic (schizophrenia, bipolar psychosis)
S = stroke, subarachnoid hemorrhage, seizures

Mnemonics got Robert through medical school, and this one was his favorite. He went over each of these possible causes and crossed out the ones that obviously didn't apply to Francine.

Though he and Mel had scoffed a bit at Dr. Valentine's tendency to overtest, Robert now found himself grateful for the doctor's thoroughness with Francine. Her brain imaging was normal, which told him the cause was not a bleed or a tumor. The lumbar puncture was normal, ruling out infection. The EEG ruled out a seizure, the MRI a stroke, and the blood work seemed to rule out everything else: electrolyte problems, uremia, thyroid storm.

Robert gulped the last of his drink and browsed through the chart again. He was left with one choice.

Other drugs.

Though the toxicology report had been normal, there were hundreds of drugs the screen wouldn't pick up.

But Mel had said he found no empty pill bottles lying around.

Why did he think to look?

Robert's head started to throb again from the rifle butt blow he'd received that morning, and his lower back felt like drying cement from his fall from the tree. He splashed some more mezcal in his glass, rolled into his hammock, placed his notebook on his chest, and started going over every chemical he could think of that could cause Francine's condition.

Tylenol, aspirin, valproic acid, lead …

He shut his eyes and pictured Francine in her ICU bed. He pictured her monitor and then—he couldn't help it—he pictured Sharon sitting at her bedside.

Now his groggy vision grew clearer, and he watched Sharon leaning watchfully over Francine's inert form.

No doubt trying to piece together on her own what had brought Francine to such a state.

A pre-sleep warmth began to suffuse Robert's torso as his mind's eye watched Sharon at work, going beyond the call of duty as she so often did.

He yawned.

His eyes fluttered shut.

His breathing slowed.

As sleep took hold of his body, his brain started to spin out new connections, blazing a chemical highway from the jungles of his hippocampus to the cognitive capital of his prefrontal cortex, assembling the new information into sensibility. His dreaming parts began blending colors, mixing cement, and revving engines in an attempt to put the pieces of this jigsaw puzzle together.

To an outside observer Robert looked perfectly still, as comatose as Francine—but under his skull was the same creative action that allowed Shakespeare to compose his sonnets.

Sound and sight asleep, Robert's mind hit REM.

The rapid eye movements meant the lights were coming up in the theater of his optic neurons, rewiring brain connections in learning curves and camera angles, sparking interest in his inner spectator as the curtains parted on his self-serving, self-reflecting dream. In his mind's eye Robert now saw Sharon. Her smile was so radiant that it lit up the ICU room where she sat by Francine, also beautiful but cold and motionless as alabaster.

Robert began to float. He didn't want to leave this room because it held Sharon, but he needed to see the other patients.

For some reason they all had altered mental status.

He floated down the hall, slapping aside leaves from an absurdly overgrown potted plant, and he glided to a landing by the bed of a man in pajamas who looked at him and raved, "*La flecha es un bisturí.*"

The arrow is a scalpel.

Robert bent to examine the wild-eyed man, who perseverated the phrase. He had a pressure dressing around his scalp. Robert carefully unwrapped the gauze and noted what looked like a bullet wound overlying the man's temporal lobe.

Traumatic intracranial bleed.

He couldn't float to the next room but used some wiring hanging from the hall ceiling to swing into it.

In that bed was an elderly Asian woman with shaking hands that looked like a bloated version of Dr. Fox.

"Help me!" she slurred at him like a drunkard. "*Mi páncreas se pudre con parásitos.*"

My pancreas rots with parasites.

Robert leaned over and prodded her liver. Her breath reeked. Syrupy and musty.

Diabetic ketoacidosis.

The demented patient in the next bed suddenly sat up and began speaking gibberish in a strangled voice that moved only one side of his mouth. "Not Thursday, nowhere here, Brooklyn words no sleep ..."

Wernicke's aphasia. Massive stroke.

Robert left the room, eager to get back to Sharon and feel the warmth of her smile. He was back on solid ground now and he hurried back to Francine's room, dodging staff and equipment.

But Sharon was no longer smiling. She was pointing at Francine's hand, shaking her head.

Robert grew more confused.

Why was she pointing there?

The knuckle on Francine's left ring finger was swollen. The rest of the hand was mottled. There were shards of shattered mirror beside it.

Robert looked at the monitor. Francine's blood pressure was low, yet her heart rate was normal. Sharon seemed unfazed by the obvious pallor of Francine's extremities, which signified impending multiorgan failure—disseminated intravascular coagulopathy.

Even though Sharon was no physician, she should know this.

Without looking at him, Sharon just kept pointing at Francine's ring finger.

What am I missing?

Robert woke with a start. He was sweating. The hut was bright. From the position of the sun, he guessed he had slept six hours.

He curled his lips into a gloating smile.

He knew Francine's diagnosis.

CHAPTER 24

Robert was impressed to find Mel shooting arrows into targets twenty yards away.

The old man learns quickly.

Three kids continued to encourage Mel's efforts, running to fetch his arrows for him. Compared to the raucous high spirits of his first crowd, they had a quieter, more businesslike energy—though still infused with a hushed excitement.

Mel focused on an old red bandanna the kids had stuck on a tree trunk. Robert watched him take a deep, easy breath.

He's in a state of flow.

Mel drew the string back, shifted his arm slightly, then released the arrow.

Right through the heart of the red.

The kids whispered a chorus of *Si!*

"Great shot, boss."

Mel whipped his head around and saw Robert. "It's all because of you—giving me good orders on how to shoot this thing."

"You've been practicing this whole time?"

"You insane? With Maja's food around?"

"I guess you're getting to like it here," Robert said.

"I like feeling alive. Strange, huh? I love how wild it is here. And these little amigos are not bad companions." He rubbed the tallest kid's hair.

The kid immediately pulled off Mel's hat and rubbed his bald head. Mel snatched the hat back, laughing.

"Now you get why it's my second home." Robert took the bow from Mel and handed it to the grinning kid. "Let's take a walk, boss."

"Something tells me you've figured out what's wrong with Francine," Mel said, his tone anxious. "Please tell me your first hunch was right. Tell me my wife is going to be okay. Please tell me Francine's diagnosis isn't fatal."

"She's going to be fine," Robert said. "What Francine's got isn't fatal."

"Oh good." Mel looked up at the sky. His eyes filled with tears. "I'm so relieved! God, my heart is jumping all over the place."

They began making a small loop around the village. Robert looked around at the familiar village sites with a sharper attention than usual, feeling pangs of nostalgia.

"How did you figure out her diagnosis?" Mel asked, his voice wary but hopeful.

"Let's just call it intuition," Robert said.

"Your intuition's a human miracle. People are still buzzing about how you diagnosed Francine's last illness."

"Her subacute bacterial endocarditis? I remember."

"Despite her atypical presentation."

"That was easy compared to this."

It was late afternoon. Twigs snapped crisply under their feet. Wildly colored parrots flapped overhead, and chirping insects wove a pulsing sine wave into the jungle surround sound.

At a clearing by the edge of the village, they stopped. Robert stared right at Mel. "Okay, before we start, I want to ask you a few questions."

"What? Sure, yeah. Ask me anything."

"Did you tell Francine about the affair?"

"I couldn't bear to tell her," Mel muttered. "I was ashamed! I'm still ashamed."

"Did you tell anyone at work about the affair?"

"Of course not!" Mel looked offended. "No one knew. I'm not completely dumb. I know how to be discreet."

"Are you kidding me? I'm sure just about everyone knew around there. You know how hospital talk goes."

Looking unnerved, Mel shook his head. "Not about this."

"Okay, then, answer me one last question. Did you really believe Francine had hurt her knuckle at the gym?"

"What does that matter?"

"Say she didn't hurt the knuckle at the gym," Robert said. "Let's say she hurt it about the same time you began the affair, right?"

"I'm not following you, Robert."

"Do you really think it was an accident that the lost wedding picture reappeared when you found Francine comatose? The glass cracked with her wedding ring next to it?"

There was a long silence. A gusty wind started shaking the canopied greenery above them in a mournful calypso. Drops fell from the wet leaves onto their faces.

"What are you saying?" Mel asked quietly.

"You tell me."

"She cracked her knuckle on the picture?"

"How long ago?"

"Same time it disappeared. When I started the affair."

"Yes."

There was a beat of silence. "She knew."

"It was a message, Mel. A love note, a real dark one."

Mel's face turned a sickly shade of yellow. Robert had never seen his old boss so distressed.

"Shit!" Mel wiped his eyes angrily. "Fuck! Goddamn it."

Robert didn't say anything.

"It was a suicide attempt," Mel said. "Francine tried to kill herself."

Robert nodded but kept quiet.

"I think something in me must've suspected it. That's why I did the tox screen, but it came back as blank as everything else. Damn it!" More tears sprang from Mel's eyes. These he didn't bother to wipe away.

Robert lowered his voice. "You said she started acting real tired around the same time, didn't you?"

"That's right," Mel said, his voice cracking.

"Wasn't getting enough sleep?"

"Even with the sleeping pills—" Mel said, his eyes suddenly widening. "Oh God, no. Wait a minute … the Ambien."

"It must be."

"She started not taking it. Saving up the pills. Hating me a little more every night she lay there not sleeping. Planning to leave me. Thinking I didn't love her."

"You loved her, but you didn't love her right."

"So she's in a prolonged sleep. There's little risk of death?"

"Technically," Robert explained, "unless there's a coingestion or comorbidity."

"Ambien doesn't show up on urine toxicology screens, right?"

"Not even the extended release kind she had."

"So she chokes down many moons worth of caps, and because she's diabetic, she probably has some degree of gastroparesis."

"Which means her gut isn't moving what's in there as fast as it should," Robert explained, "leading to prolonged altered mental status. The fact that she's still alive and that all the imaging studies, EEG, and other blood tests have been normal means that she'll be fine. Her body hasn't gone into organ failure. Although she's in a stupor, she's maintaining her airway and oxygenating. I wouldn't be surprised if she's awake by now. My intuition tells me that she's going to be okay. Time takes care of Ambien just fine."

"You must be right!" Mel yelled, and lunged into a big bear hug with Robert, his cheeks streaming with tears. "Robert, you saved me. I'm living again. Because she's going to be fine!" Mel pulled back, holding both of Robert's shoulders, looking at him in total seriousness. "Anything ... you ever want, Robert. *Any*thing! I'm good for it."

"I know you are," Robert said. "And I do want something from you. When you see her, I want you to apologize to her. Tell her you're an idiot and tell her how much you love her. Then start showing that love in a way that respects her space and gives her all the attention and help and company she wants—and none of it she doesn't want. So that next time I see you two I'll feel comfortable hanging with you both. I'll like it. That's what you can do for me."

"If she by some miracle still wants to be with me, that's exactly what I'll do. I'll make this better. All this time she's been gone from me, I've learned how much I want to do that more than anything."

"Good," Robert said, believing him. "I'm glad to hear that."

"Okay then." Mel dropped his arms and his gaze. They had almost circled around to where they left the village.

"I have to go hunt for dinner now, Mel. Want to go grab your bow and arrow and help?"

"Not really. Not now." Mel wiped the tears off his face, smiling. "I'm going to pack. Then I'm going to see Guillermo. I'm going to thank him for his endearing hospitality."

CHAPTER 25

Robert brought back a slew of wild turkeys for the village and dropped them off with Maja, who said Mel and Guillermo were with the prisoner. This surprised Robert, and he hurried to the detention hut. He found them inside, going through Fox's medicine bag. Fox was staring daggers at them, but the fresh strip of tape over his mouth saved them from his grating voice and noxious insults.

"Ah, the hunter is home from the hunt," Mel said, as Robert came in.

"Good," Guillermo said. "We need arbitration."

Robert joined them before a table spread with what they'd been pulling from Fox's bag.

"Mel has a pretty far out theory about this stuff," Guillermo explained.

"It's not a theory, Gil," Mel said. "I'd stake my reputation on it."

Robert almost laughed at Mel's nickname for Guillermo and waited for Guillermo to explode in protest. But Guillermo just looked more serious than ever and said, "That's not good enough."

"What are we looking at here?" Robert asked.

"Transplant gear," Mel said.

"So he claims." Guillermo picked up a plastic vial. "How can you know something like that for sure?"

"I did a surgery residency."

"I thought you never finished the residency," Guillermo said.

"I got grandfathered into emergency medicine after I graduated, but while I was doing surgery I thought I'd go into organ transplant. I loved the challenge of placing another person's organs and tricking the host body into accepting it. What could be cooler than that? But then my daughter was born, and I knew I couldn't be a surgeon and have any kind of family life. So I finished my residency and worked my way up from an urgent-care center to ER administration. Gave up chasing the surgeon dream, but I keep up with the literature. Hell, I still read the *Annals of Surgery* in the bathroom. I know my transplant-surgery medications."

Guillermo shook the vial gently. "And you're saying this is for posttransplant patients?"

"Damn right. That's an immune suppressor."

"Is he right, Robert?" Guillermo asked.

"It's possible." Robert rummaged through what was left in Fox's bag. There were vials of antibiotics and morphine, vasopressors for blood pressure control, and other medications.

"Why don't we just ask Dr. Fox?" Robert suggested.

Guillermo and Mel both looked at Robert, irritated. "The guy won't say anything," Mel explained.

"Just keeps saying they told him to bring this stuff, but he doesn't know why," Guillermo said. "I'd be glad to shovel some hot embers down his pants to get him to talk more."

Robert walked over to Fox and ripped the tape off his mouth.

"You don't feed me," Fox immediately spluttered. "You gag me, you go through my things, you slap me around, you …"

"Dr. Fox," Robert said, raising his hand. Fox shut up, but continued to glare. "The stuff in your bag. Is it for organ transplantation? Kidney transplants?"

"It's for when we get you on the operating table." A malignant gleam flared in Fox's eyes. "For keeping you awake when we take out your liver and heart and show it to you still pulsing. And for when we slice off the top of that old man's cranium like a soft-boiled egg and replace his cerebellum with fatty tissue we suction from the babbling blimp over there."

"It's for taking out livers, isn't it?" Robert asked patiently.

"I cure livers, I don't steal them," Fox shot back indignantly. "I told you, I deal with liver disease, which occasionally means resection of lobes. You're an ignorant …"

Robert put the tape back over the man's mouth, and turned to Guillermo. "He's right. Those are all surgical medications."

"Except for the Azathioprine," Guillermo said.

"Yeah," Robert said, "but that's used for ulcerative colitis …"

"And transplant surgeries," Mel shot back. "Particularly kidney transplants."

"Let's assume Mel is right," Robert said. "What do we do?"

"Always start with what you know," Guillermo said. "Fox is a hepatologist who's here with a bunch of other specialists."

"Maybe it's to help with surgeries in remote villages," Robert said.

"I don't buy it," Guillermo said. "Narcotraficantes care only about themselves and big bucks."

"And those other doctors," Robert said. "Why are the narcos bringing all these specialists to Kundal?"

They sat in silence for a moment, thinking.

Mel's face suddenly drained of blood and he made a sound like something had just ruptured in his lower belly.

"What?" Robert asked.

"The girls they kidnapped. Maybe they're not selling them as sex slaves. Maybe they're …"

"Taking their organs," Guillermo whispered.

"But it doesn't make sense," Mel said. "Kundal's kind of—no offense, Gil—kind of backward, no? Hardly a place for that kind of modern surgery."

"On the other hand, Kundal is by the coast," Robert mused. "A good place to transport organs out by boat without raising suspicions."

"And the hundreds of villages around there have plenty of young healthy kids ripe for the taking," Guillermo said. "Damn, *that's* what they've been doing these last months. That's been the fever in my bones. The narcos have paid off the officials in Guatemala City to close down Kundal so they can set up their bloodsucking work. They've moved on from drugs and sex to organs."

"How could they perform transplant surgeries in the open jungle?" Mel asked. "Even with the personnel and the equipment and the drugs. They need operating rooms."

Robert grew pensive for a moment, then heard a muffled but familiar tune. Fox started humming behind his tape. Robert's face flushed as he realized it was a song popular lately in Guatemala called "*Toma Mi Corazon.*" He hustled angrily over to Fox. "So we're right? You're here to take organs?" Fox made his humming louder, his eyes dancing with sickening humor.

Robert knocked him unconscious with one punch.

"Damn, Robert!" Mel said, aghast. "Don't you like music?"

"The title of that song translates to 'Take My Heart,'" Guillermo said solemnly.

"Oh," Mel said. "I guess he's telling us we're right."

"Your question is still on the table," Guillermo said.

"Where's the operating theater for this medical terrorism?" Robert asked an unconscious Fox.

"Jungle's a terrible place for surgery," Mel went on. "Insects, monkeys, birds, all sorts of animals everywhere. Dirt, scat, moss, leaves, trees ..."

"They're doing it underground," Guillermo said, between clenched teeth.

Robert groaned as Guillermo's insight hit home. "Of course! The cenotes."

"Cenotes?" Mel repeated.

"The underground limestone caves in Kundal. Any one of them would make an ideal operating space. Cool, clean, and sterile as any operating room in the U.S."

"And near the coast, like you say," Guillermo said. "Extract every bright red organ from the kid, throw the shell away, load the goods in coolers and sail them anywhere in the world."

Robert felt Guillermo's acid bitterness eating away at his own gut. He started pacing and fuming in the small confines of the prison hut, his growing fury tempting him to run through the walls. "Probably truckloads of kids there now, underground prisoners, writhing with claustrophobia as they get strapped down for evisceration. Assembly-line evisceration."

"Motherfuckers!" Guillermo marched toward Fox, cupped the prisoner's jaw with one hand and crossed his other hand to the side of the man's head, ready to twist and break his neck.

"No!" Robert and Mel yelled in unison. Together they sprang at Guillermo and yanked his hands apart.

"Let go of me!" Guillermo roared, looking half-crazed. But Robert's enormous strength, combined with Mel's added bulk, kept him from the prisoner.

"Think of the headline, Gil!" Mel yelled. "'American Surgeon Caught in Organ Traffic Scandal!'"

Guillermo stopped fighting but his body still quivered. "That could get the whole world down here to help us." His voice trembled with suppressed rage.

"We get him to Guatemala City," Mel went on. "Get him locked up, I call my press contacts, including the foreign editor of *The New York Times*."

Guillermo's body started to relax as the sense of Mel's idea sunk in.

Soon Robert and Mel were able to bring Guillermo back to the table. They all sat in silence staring at Fox's equipment, which seemed to have a malevolent sheen.

"Call your press guys now." With a disgusted look, Guillermo gingerly picked up a scalpel as if it were one of Satan's long-nailed fingers.

"Soon as we get in range of the city," Mel said. "No reception here."

More silence.

Guillermo whirled and threw the scalpel straight into Fox's calf, where it embedded with a soft thud. A red bloom stained his trouser leg. Fox jerked and moaned but didn't wake up.

Mel and Robert just blinked.

"That'll make it harder for him to run away from you guys," Guillermo said.

Robert quietly went and grabbed some bandages from the supply closet. “You’re going to Kundal, then?” He pulled out the scalpel and set about stanching Fox’s wound.

“I have to.” Guillermo stood up and straightened his clothes. “There must be dozens of innocent kids there. I have to save them.”

“I’m going with you,” Robert said.

“Mel can’t handle Fox by himself,” Guillermo said. “I’ll be fine, Robert. I’ve been doing this for a long time.”

“You’re not doing this on your own,” Robert repeated.

“You don’t want any of this, Robert. There are going to be a lot of bad guys at Kundal. I can’t guarantee that you’d come out alive. You might not go home to those soft arms you live for.”

“Look, Guillermo.” Robert finished his wrapping job and stood to face his mentor. “Your words hurt me, and the fact that you don’t want me around is devastating. But I know you’re trying to protect me, whether or not you admit it. You’re right. I want to be with Sharon more than I want to be here.”

Guillermo shook his head and looked away.

“But how can I be happy with her if I leave you alone to do this? I couldn’t live with myself, let alone her. Rimaldi let us know the score. Drug cartels are going epic with their plans here, escalating from slavery and the sex trade to strip-mining young kids of their organs. It’s enough. This is your home, Guillermo, and it’s been mine, too. It’s where I really grew up. Where I found my calling. Where I embraced karma. It’s time we take it back from these bastards and put them down.” Robert paused and smiled. “Consider it my going-away present. Our last hurrah.”

Guillermo’s dark face brightened, and Robert’s heart lifted. “As long as you know what we’re getting into.”

"I know."

"You're probably not going to make it out of here," Guillermo said. "And neither am I."

"I know," Robert repeated.

"Why don't we just wait until we get to Guatemala City?" Mel suggested. "There's no sense in going on a kamikaze mission. Once we get enough press, then the government will have to act."

"By then it'll be too late for some of these kids," Robert said. "Mel, there's no other choice."

"I can wait for you guys," Mel went on. "Make sure you get back okay. See what the story is I can tell the *Times.*"

"No," Guillermo said. "Get the story out right away, Mel. Start it rolling."

"We can handle this," Robert said. "Ernesto can help you with Fox, and you need to get back to Francine ASAP. Tomorrow morning, you're off."

There was a loud groan behind them. Fox had come awake and was feeling the deep-tissue pain in his calf.

"You feel that?" Robert called, silencing Fox's moans for a second. "That's karma coming to you and all your colleagues. And it's just the start."

PART 2

Organ Trafficking Statistics:

- *Although more than 120,000 patients need healthy organs in the United States, there are only about twenty thousand donors annually. On average, twenty people die each day from a lack of available transplants.*[7]

- *One organ is sold illegally somewhere on the globe every hour.*[8]

- *Ten percent of all transplants are performed illegally.*[9]

- *Patients often pay up to $200,000 for a single kidney to gangs who harvest organs from vulnerable, desperate people, who get paid as little as $5,000 (if they're not otherwise having their organs being taken by force).*[10]

- *To get the illegal organs onto airplanes, mules (i.e., organ transporters who are not medically trained) will wrap them in plastic and tape them to their stomachs, or will place them in hollowed-out objects such as basketballs or coconuts. The organs are not stored at the temperatures recommended by the American Academy of Surgeons and often end up with some sort of defect upon arrival into the United States or another first-world country.*[11]

---

7 *American Transplant Foundation, "Facts and Myths."*

8 *World Health Organization, "The State of the International Organ Trade."*

9 *United Nations Global Initiative to Fight Human Trafficking, "Trafficking for Organ Trade."*

10 *Denis Campbell and Nicola Davison. "Illegal Kidney Trade Books." The Guardian, May 27, 2012.*

11 *World Health Organization, "Illicit Organ Trafficking and the Black Market for Human Body Parts."*

CHAPTER 26

Robert and Guillermo rose the next day before the sun, packed their supplies, gathered their weapons, and headed out of the village just as Maja lit the breakfast fire.

"Tear their heads off and scatter their bones," she called as they passed, not bothering to keep her voice down.

"She enjoys alarming everyone out of bed," Guillermo said, giving her a large formal wave.

Robert smiled and blew her a kiss, and she blew one right back with a smack loud enough to startle a rare quetzal bird into undulating flight. The morning smelled of fresh dew and pitaya vines.

To evade trafficker guards, they avoided all trails and wrangled and hacked their way through thick brush without saying a word.

After an hour, they took a water break by a cluster of massive Ceiba trees, both of them sweating but their breath strong and steady.

"Black widow on your neck." Guillermo reached over to flick it off.

"Thanks," Robert said, matter-of-factly.

"Now we're even for when you stopped me from stepping on that copperhead."

Robert took a swig of water and wiped his forehead. "If Fox is their only liver guy, good chance they've sent out a hunting party for him."

"We could use that if they ambush us. You look so much like him, just pretend you're him. Could buy us the time we need to get our weapons going."

"I guess," Robert said. "But if they know I'm lying they'll kill me on the spot."

Guillermo nodded, glugged down some water, wiped his mouth, and eyed some plants in the brush. "I spent a good part of my childhood in Kundal, you know." He leaned down and studied the leaves, took a handful of berries, gave Robert half, and tossed the rest into his own mouth.

The skins had a bitter green taste, but when split a delicious citrus-blueberry taste wiped out the sting.

"What part of your childhood?" Robert accepted another mouthful of berries from his medicine-man mentor.

"After the narcos invaded and killed my family." Guillermo chewed thoughtfully. "I didn't have a place to go. I remember walking right into the jungle, half-hoping I'd meet up with a jaguar or leopard. I imagined ripping some savage animal like that limb from limb with my mighty rage. But I think I was half-hoping to die and thought I might as well go out having an adventure I could tell my parents about in the happy hunting grounds when we'd meet again. Fortunately, the feral cats ignored me, and I ended up stumbling upon Kundal. Can you imagine? Terrified kid after such a traumatic experience coming upon that serene marvel, a glorious Mayan city, hidden for centuries and still unknown to most of the world."

"I can see it," Robert said. "Probably had invisible strings coming out of the main temple hooked into your navel."

"I don't know about that." Guillermo smiled, pleased with the idea. "Who knows? The truth is always deeper than the senses."

Their heads turned at the sound of a ruckus behind them. A team of guinea hens came squawking and pecking out of the brush into their small clearing.

"Good morning, fellows." At the sound of Guillermo's gentle but resonant voice, they stopped dead and quieted. Then just as abruptly they started squawking and milling around again, pecking at the ground with their small heads and waddling around with their big fat bodies.

"They're like a gang of grouchy teenagers," Robert said.

Guillermo nodded.

The birds went right through the berry bush on to the brush beyond, searching for ground bugs and seeds. Their irregular bursts of shrieking and quiet clucking faded into the vibrant wall of ambient jungle noise.

"Actually, there was something kind of mystical about that first night in Kundal." Guillermo's dark eyes brightened with the memory. "I climbed a high tower with crumbling bricks and spaced notches for my bare feet and hands. I scrambled until I reached this platform at the top, where I could see the whole layout of the ruins and a carpet of treetops lit by a bright moon and stars. I felt like I was in a rocket ship. Peaceful night lights, quiet, gentle breeze, and I had a pocketful of these berries."

Guillermo paused and popped three more into his mouth. He chewed slowly, as if the taste were the memory itself.

"Odd," he finally said, "how good I felt up there. A helpless little boy, alone, my brain seared by the awful murders of my parents. I felt they were still alive somehow in me, wanting me not to collapse with the horror, wanting me to get above it any way I could. And I was above it. I was above everything in that tower."

Guillermo shook his head. Robert waited for him to speak again.

"I was getting some strange stuff up there, something from where death and life connect. Just that morning, my parents were brutally murdered, my village destroyed, my whole world gone like a dream a minute after you wake up. Maybe I was radically disoriented from shock and hunger. But, spread out below me, the whole jungle felt friendly, like it was extending open arms. And it whispered. The whispers of the night jungle, shushing me, calming me, saying, 'We'll take care of you, we're watching.' When I fell asleep, it was like falling into the immenseness of nature, how space and everything in it spread farther than I could think, and I was nestled in the middle of it, as safe and fixed as the center of a circle, the tiniest point perfectly placed in the largest sphere imaginable. Nothing could dislodge me, nothing could hurt me anymore. Nature was the home I had been away from, but now I'd returned and it was taking care of me. Amazing, huh? This jungle. Nature."

Robert nodded but didn't know what to say. He was uncharacteristically moved. It was the same lesson his mother had infused in him as a child, and hearing Guillermo's fatherly tones made her presence feel as real to Robert as the sound of the fluttering leaves around them.

Hear how the wind brings the tree alive? How well you breathe, darling, is how well you live.

"And now they want to take over this jungle?" Guillermo exploded. "Use it for butchery? Decimate its inhabitants? It's like they want to kill my mother and father right before my very eyes again."

He growled and took another swig of water.

His outburst jolted Robert from motherly remembrance to fierce resolve in a split second.

"The traffickers have corrupt ties in Guatemala City," Robert said. "Why don't they just rent out a surgical center there? Better conditions, better product."

"They're not concerned about organ health. As long as they can sell it for the big bucks, that's their aim. Who's going to complain if the organ fails? Who could they complain to? And not everyone in Guatemala is corrupt. Too easy for word to get out. Lots of good guys there. But here—just the trees and us."

Robert looked around and noted the thick brush, the bulky lattice of the giant trees, the impenetrable dark places pocked throughout, the dark grays and opaque greens—countless hiding places large and small beyond the reach of probing eyes and high-tech scanners. "No government agency or army could find them—if they come looking, the traffickers have a thousand perfect ambush spots. And they have massive manpower. So many goddamn psychopaths teeming into our rainforests. And the forces of law and order can't figure out how to arrest them. It almost feels like they've stopped trying. How could they give up? They should be helping us out."

"It's just us now," Guillermo said, "so we better get going."

"I hope none of those enemy scouts have been listening in on our little water-cooler chat."

"They haven't." Guillermo's confidence convinced Robert. "No one's in earshot, I can tell. But we're getting close."

They cut their own path with machetes, making quick, clean cuts for minimum noise. Guillermo paused every half-minute to attune his internal radar.

The terrain became steeper, and the two worked hard to keep up a decent pace, remaining ten yards parallel to the main path.

"A new noise," Guillermo whispered.

They halted, crouching under a low bower ablaze with red jewel-like flowers. Robert put on his high-resolution magnification glasses and scanned the upward timberline.

Blue sky. No clouds.

He looked three hundred and sixty degrees into the overhead trees.

Spider monkeys. Parrots. Woodpecker. Sleeping snake.

Barely any sun getting through.

"Nothing," Robert said under his breath.

Guillermo nodded, pointing his index finger forward.

They continued trekking up.

Guillermo halted, then pointed to one ear.

Robert heard only his thumping heart. He closed his eyes and calmed himself. He gave ear to the wind. He heard a faint, throbbing buzz, a pulsing wave of ordered activity.

Human activity.

His eyes sprang open. Guillermo pointed to a rocky ledge ahead, an overhanging cliff.

Robert nodded. Soundlessly, they sank to the ground, flattened out on their stomachs, and pulled themselves to the edge.

Robert saw the limestone Mayan temple of Kundal rising into view—seventy meters tall, surrounded by a stone plaza, weathered by the ages and flanked by three imposing buildings.

The place teemed with armed men.

"Shit," Guillermo whispered, looking woeful.

Robert shook his head. "I hope we have a plan B."

CHAPTER 27

Still lying on his stomach, Robert felt like he'd been kicked by a mule. He counted thirty-six men with guns, some milling about the open field, others manning a makeshift prison holding twenty young villagers.

Next to the prison, looking like civilians but still threatening and shady, the American physicians bustled around large tables that held computer gear and what looked like a communications setup.

And medical equipment.

Robert turned to Guillermo, who was studying the tower above the temple. "Machine guns," he murmured, shaking his head.

The temple was manned by two men almost eye level with their perch on the edge of the overhang.

They slowly inched backward out of the tower's view.

"We have to go back," Guillermo said, "get Armando and some reinforcements. Even then we'll be way outnumbered. Still underdogs."

"We can't go back, Guillermo, and you know it. Those twenty kids won't have any organs by then."

"We have to be realistic, Roberto. This is no small apartment full of your New York rapists or drunken wife-abusers. We're not going to swing down on a zip line and smash through a little window onto some lowlife zoned out in front of a television. There are three dozen armed guards who know what they're doing, some with machine guns and we don't know what else. What are we? One enthusiastic gymnast and an old man armed with slingshots."

"What's with you all of a sudden? We can't let those kids go under the knife."

Guillermo shook his head. "Too many bad guys. We can't beat them. It's too risky."

"Too risky? You're the one who taught me that one man can beat an army of a hundred if he's properly trained and uses his brain. 'One wasp,' you said, 'in a truck full of terrorists. The pilot swats at it, the truck crashes and the wasp flies away.' We're two wasps, and they're just forty-something in a truck. We can do this."

"Wasps also get smashed like flies, especially when the front seat has forty fly swatters." Guillermo stood and turned toward the trail leading back to the village. "I'm not going to be responsible for making some girl in New York a widow."

Robert's puzzled brow instantly smoothed. "Oh, that's what this is about, is it? Give it up, Guillermo. You and romantic sympathy go together like vinegar and donuts. I told you I couldn't live with myself—or Sharon—if I walked away from a killing field like this. This world may be filled with apathetic people, but you know I'm not one of them. Neither is she. Those are our people down there, and they're facing hell if we don't do something about it. If I die, Sharon will live with it. If I leave here now, I won't be able to face her. Go if you want. We came here to do a job, and I'm going to do it—with or without you."

Guillermo's gaze didn't flinch a second during Robert's tirade. Robert thought he heard a kind of applause as a sudden upwind rattled the leaves.

Guillermo smiled. "I was hoping you'd say that."

Robert smiled back. "Thought so."

"Let's work on plan B." Guillermo picked up twigs and foliage from the ground.

Robert did the same. They were in the tower guards' sightlines. They needed to camouflage their heads before they scouted the area again. Without another word, they turned their heads into leaf-and-twig masses that moved and fluttered no faster or slower than the green and brown jungle floor they slithered over on their return to the cliff edge.

Together they peered through the twitching flora hanging over their foreheads at the scene below, studying the flow of activity, getting a sense of who the leaders were, who was doing what, and what patterns emerged from the movements.

"By the radio," Guillermo whispered. "His name is Baraka. He's originally from downtown Guatemala City. Hooks village kids on heroin. Free samples. Then ropes them in. Armies of them. Goes back and forth between Guatemala City and the jungle. Wreaks havoc everywhere. Lord Baraka."

"Drug lord."

"Now turned organ lord."

"More buck for the bang."

"CFO of an empire."

Robert nodded.

Scowling, they continued to study the activity below.

"Surgeons are still unloading," Robert whispered. "Haven't started harvesting yet."

Guillermo eyed the tower and growled. One of the guards was urinating onto the ancient plaza. Robert had to restrain himself from jumping up and firing an arrow into the man's groin.

How dare he desecrate this place?

"Got a pattern." Guillermo pointed with his chin. "That surgeon. Wheeling the equipment. See? Guard leads him to that building over there. And look—coming out."

"Another guard and a surgeon ..."

"With an empty cart."

"That's the building, then. Hospital's in there."

"No," Guillermo said.

"No?"

"Not *in* there."

"*Under* there," Robert amended, understanding dawning. "The cenotes. That's where they're prepping a makeshift operating room. Cool, sterile, quiet."

"Whole labyrinth down there," Guillermo said. "Water tunnels to the coast. Perfect for transporting the organs. They're all interconnected."

Getting excited, Robert whispered, "We find one cenote, sneak in, find their operating room, kill the guards, take the kids out, outrun any pursuit, lose them in the maze."

"Too many guards. They know the tunnels. And all that firepower? One spray of bullets, one grenade, and they'll be taking *our* organs."

"Not if we kill the surgeons."

"They'd just get more. And who will stop them then if we're out of the picture?"

"The press, if Mel gets through."

Guillermo grimaced as he considered the plan. Then he relaxed. "Sun Tzu," he whispered.

"*The Art of War*," Robert said. "Okay. What about it?"

"'The highest excellence is to subdue the enemy's army without fighting at all.'"

"Come on, Guillermo. I told you I'm not leaving here without a fight!"

"We're not leaving here."

"But we're not fighting?"
"If you can't fight them ..."
"Join them?"
"You got it," Guillermo said.
"Ah," Robert said. "You mean infiltrate."
Guillermo smiled. "That's right, Dr. Fox."

CHAPTER 28

Robert and Guillermo headed back down the hill as quiet and sure-footed as a pair of stalking panthers. Soon they found a place to circle back toward the temple grounds.

They came as close as they dared, looking for a hiding spot where Guillermo could park with their archery and gun gear and keep a ready lookout on any stir Robert caused.

The plan was rough and risky, but Robert was itching to put it into action. He figured his two-day beard could blur any big differences between his face and Dr. Fox's.

Fox had said none of the doctors knew each other, barely looked at each other.

Each probably felt some basic shame.

Robert planned to act like the bedraggled hepatologist, lost in the mayhem of yesterday's gun battle, who finally found his way back to camp. He'd play dumb and disoriented, figure out what he was up against, either recruit or silence the other surgeons, depending. At night, when everyone else slept, he and Guillermo would wipe out what needed wiping out and save whomever needed saving.

Again, extremely risky.

And the moment any of them saw through his act, Robert was a dead man.

Have to be a good actor. Have to feel the part.

Feel disoriented. Tainted by shame.

Guillermo led the way, looking for a good spot, moving confidently to some place he had in mind.

Probably remembered Kundal from when he was a lost boy and found himself here. He knows where he's going.

Being so keyed up in such a sacred place, Robert couldn't stop images of Mayan culture flooding his mind as he followed in Guillermo's sure footsteps. He'd always been awed by the Mayans and had immersed himself in reading about them during college. It was one of the reasons he decided to come to Guatemala as a medical student.

Great warriors.

Even better scholars.

Their advances in writing, architecture, and mathematics still have scientists shaking their heads.

Robert always found it galling how poorly modern people in general understood ancient wisdom. Despite centuries of translations and redactions, they insisted on taking everything they read literally, missing the powerful associative impact.

So many of those sacred stories had connections with medicine, even those in the Old Testament.

The Noah story.

Forty days and forty nights.

The same amount of time it takes for a fractured bone to heal, or a broken heart to start mending.

Six weeks.

Took me that long to get moving after my mother and brother died.

Robert remembered the branch that started knocking against his bedroom window at his grandfather's house, making him jump from his bed where he'd been sunk in depression. Staring at the branch, Robert had realized that the wind had animated it, and he remembered his mother's words about how the wind makes the trees alive. He had found himself gulping lung-filling breaths like a man coming out of the desert at a drinking fountain.

The air was delicious.

Heaven-sent.

Earthbound.

And Robert could sense at that moment how his mother wanted him to live again, to remember her from then on as a source of goodness in his life, not a depressant.

Forty days.

No dove at his window, and the branch wasn't an olive branch.

But the clouds were gone from his head.

Sacrifice.

Giving up something you want for something you need.

Robert remembered how his own mind opened up on reading the prophet Isaiah's words.

No more sacrificial offerings. The blood of bulls and goats revolts me.

Search for justice. Help the oppressed.

Robert grew from sacrifice. He had put himself through college, working full-time with a full course load and disciplining his body with martial arts every night while so many other students were drinking, partying, and having sex they couldn't remember the next day.

Sacrificing even here, right now, giving up going home to Sharon and putting my life on the line.

"Get your head out of the clouds, Roberto. This is the spot," Guillermo whispered, waving his hand in front of Robert's face. They had stopped.

As Robert snapped back to the present, a phrase echoed in the canyons of his mind like a shouted Mayan prayer.

We are all children of the sun.

He shook his head, clearing the cobwebs.

Lemon sunlight infiltrated the heavy limbs above them, painting vibrant pools of brightness on the forest floor.

Robert took a deep breath and looked around. They were on a hill covered by lush vegetation, with an optimal view of the main temple. With their spy equipment, Guillermo would have a commanding view of everything going on there.

"It's perfect, Guillermo."

"It'll do. And it's close enough for you to scramble back, if that becomes necessary."

"And high enough for us to fight off any assault."

"Look at this. Special treat." Guillermo took two steps and carefully put his hands on what looked like a large bush with spiky inch-long thorns.

And pulled it free.

"*Voila.*"

There was a large opening on the ground with a descending limestone staircase.

"Goddamn!" Robert said in a hushed tone.

"Goes right into the underground cenotes," Guillermo said, his eyes eager and bright. "I spent countless hours when I was a lost boy, roaming around in there. I chipped arrow signs in every wall down there, showing how to get back to this escape hatch. Remember that."

"Got it." Robert stripped himself of his weapons and any gear a disoriented hepatologist would never have. He didn't enjoy separating himself from his beloved Sig Sauer or the two Navy SEAL ankle knives, but he did. He'd probably be searched thoroughly before they let him inside the camp.

Sacrifice.

A few minutes later, he was ready.

Robert stared at Guillermo, who seemed to hesitate.

"What's wrong?" Robert asked.

"I got a bad feeling."

"Too bad."

"Everything's been going well so far," Guillermo said.

Robert nodded. There was always something unnerving when a plan seemed to fall into place so easily. "Stick to the plan, right? Isn't that what you taught me?"

"Some plan. Go in there and kill everybody."

"Just the ones that need it."

"I got a bad feeling."

"See you later." Robert ignored the voice inside reminding him that when Guillermo had a bad feeling it meant trouble ahead. He started to hyperventilate like a mad man, letting his eyes go wild. Guillermo gave him a violent shove, and he stumbled out of their hideaway.

And staggered toward the temple like someone hallucinating.

CHAPTER 29

After three steps, Robert spied an oozing marsh patch and flopped into it. He ripped his clothes, took off his shoes, and rubbed himself with the mossy sludge, griming his scalp and face until he resembled someone who had barely survived a mudslide. Then, as if in a daze, he got to his feet and lurched toward the camp, weaving and waving like a drunk.

The two armed guards at the entrance scowled at his approach. When Robert got close enough, he stopped, bent over with both hands on his knees, and panted. Both guards were overbulked with muscle.

"Park is closed," one said.

"For repairs," the other said.

"Turn around," the first said.

"Go back to your tour group."

"Do I look like a fucking tourist?" Robert raved in his best Southern accent.

His outburst instantly changed their expressions from dopey to hyper, and their hands went right to their holstered guns.

"Excuse me, amigo?"

"You want to eat this," the second guard said, pulling out his gun and aiming it at Robert's nose. "Back off and quiet down!"

It took every ounce of acting skill Robert could muster not to whip the gun out of the thug's hand and pistol-whip him upside the head with it. Instead, he stumbled back a step, assumed a timid, cowed face, and raised his hands as if in surrender to their commanding presences.

"No, no, no," he whined. "Please, I'm supposed to be with my group. I was taken here by a bunch of soldiers. I'm a surgeon. There was a shooting."

The two men looked at each other. As far as Robert could see, nothing passed between them. They stared back at Robert.

Eyes still empty.

"Oh, yeah?" the first guard said. "Says who?"

"The surgeons," Robert said. "I'm American. I'm a hepatologist."

"Snake doctor?" the gun-happy one asked.

"No, that's a herpetologist." Robert acted like he was still trying to catch his breath. "I'm a liver doctor, a surgeon who does transplants. The liver … it's here." Robert pointed to the right upper quadrant of his abdomen. "The organ? The liver organ?"

"Ah," the first guard said. "Organ guy, another organ doctor." He whacked his partner on the arm. Robert flinched as the whack made the partner's trigger finger twitch slightly. "Put your gun away. He's one of the organ guys."

"There was one missing," the guard said. "One organ doctor missing. They told us. They told us to look for … a …" and at this he patted his pockets until he found a slip of paper, which he took out and squinted at, then looked at Robert. "*Un doctor del hígado*," he said. "What kind of doctor did you say you were?"

"A liver surgeon," Robert said, holding back his desire to beat both men to a bloody pulp.

"Liver doctor, that's right," the gunman said, double-checking the slip of paper.

"We have a picture, too, don't we?" the other guard said, pulling out a driver's license photo of Dr. Fox.

Both guards crowded around the picture, looking back and forth from it to Robert.

"What's your name?"

"Verne Fox," Robert said.

"Okay," the guard wielding the gun said. "Follow me and don't try anything funny or we blow you apart. You got that?"

Robert nodded respectfully.

The guard gestured to Robert to follow. A few minutes later they emerged from the narrow entrance opening into the main temple square.

Robert liked the fact that there were unknown or little-known Mayan temples throughout Guatemala. The splendor of the Kundal ruins he'd seen only through binoculars rose powerfully before his eyes. Even under these strained circumstances, it filled the air with an aura of wisdom and power, and Robert tried to absorb it without losing focus.

The ruins, some still covered by vegetation, splayed with monuments and statues of Mayan gods.

The pair of massive pyramid temples flanking an ancient square.

The limestone high tower.

The guard led him to the communication table—a stone slab shaded by a dark-green sun tarp. Saluting briskly, he halted before a young cigar-smoker, who sat in a rusting lawn chair doing work. Baraka stood a few feet away, scrutinizing the activities of the prisoners.

"Sir," the guard said.

The cigar-smoker squinted up from his pile of computer parts and paperwork. "Cool it with the *sir* crap, would you? Who's this?"

"Missing surgeon," the guard barked, standing at attention.

"Hepatologist," Robert said.

"Ah, the liver man," Baraka said, turning around. He then addressed the guard. "Better get back to Juan before he gets lost standing in front of the entrance."

"Yes, sir." The guard clicked his heels, pivoted, nearly fell, then marched away.

"So hard to get good help these days," Baraka said laconically.

Baraka was a compact, six-foot man. His clothes were casual but perfectly tailored: a long-sleeved charcoal T-shirt, aerodynamic running pants, and what Robert recognized as Prada sneakers. His face was massive and pockmarked, with downward-slanting eyebrows that created a large, ponderous furrow right above his nose, as if he were ready to lash out at anything that disturbed him.

He fixed Robert with his predator stare. The cigar-smoker cleared his throat nervously, rustled through the papers, and shoved one of them at Baraka. Baraka looked at it, not happy with what he read. "Where have you been, Fox?"

Through the haze of cigar smoke, Robert saw Baraka's poison-sac eyes lining him up.

Best not play around with this guy.

"We were ambushed," he said, acting exasperated. "Scared me shitless. I'm a doctor, not a soldier. I just ran and ran, even before I knew I was running. I got completely lost. I couldn't hear any more shots. Lucked my way here, thank God. I'm starving and thirsty and tired, but I want to get to work and then head back home. This is not what I signed up for. You got surgery tools I can use?"

"You brought them, you should know." Baraka's gaze remained on Robert.

"I'm hoping they weren't stolen by those bandits," Robert responded.

There was a sudden outburst of terrible screaming and all heads whipped around. Two guards had entered the prison cage ten yards away and had taken hold of an adolescent boy. The other young prisoners were shouting at the guards, one of whom silenced them by spraying machine gun fire over their heads. The deafening sound faded into racking sobs and whimpers, but the boy they had grabbed kept yelling and fighting. The machine-gunner grabbed the boy's hair and pressed the smoking gun barrel against the kid's cheek, searing his flesh. The boy's yells turned to the wails of someone in agony, and the kid crumpled, cries ripping from his lungs.

Baraka watched Robert carefully. "Damn teenagers don't respect their elders."

Robert's heart thumped violently against his chest. He had to restrain himself from going on a rampage.

Revenge is going to be sweet.

"To help pay my way through medical school, I worked in a slaughterhouse." Robert shrugged. "Same kind of bawling and squealing I used to hear there."

"Funny," Baraka said, "doesn't say anything about that on your bio."

"Bet it doesn't say much about my prom date with Dana Marie Tanner, either," Robert said. "Doesn't mean I didn't give her a roofie."

Baraka kept on glaring, then his face broke into a smile and he guffawed. "I bet you did," he said, mimicking Robert's drawl.

"His first surgery is in thirty minutes," the cigar-smoker said.

"Okay, Fox," Baraka said. "We'll get some food to you and, meanwhile, take a fucking shower. You look like the loser in a pig fight, and you smell even worse. Graucho!" he yelled, and a somber bearded guard trotted over. "Take him to the temple. This is Dr. Fox. His name should be on a hammock there with his schedule."

The guard nodded and led Robert across the square to one of the temples. On the way, Robert counted thirty guards, stationed at the area's perimeter. The kid with the seared face was curled in a fetal ball, holding his hands to his face; a younger girl knelt beside him. The whole cage of young victims was a cramped arena of misery and despair. To see all that vibrant youth dispirited and broken stoked Robert's inner fires to a roar, but he kept his outward mood calm and nonchalant, as if such atrocity were par for the course of his jaded life.

The guard brought him into the doorway of the first temple.

"Gracias," Robert murmured, and the guard left without another sound. Robert walked in, and a man and a woman in scrubs looked up from where they stood rubbing sanitizer into their hands and on their arms.

Getting ready for surgery.

"Hey." Robert made his way to a hammock with a clipboard in it.

"Damn," the woman said, "you smell like a bowel resection."

"I'm cardiovascular, and she's general surgery," the man said.

"I'm hepatology." Robert picked up the clipboard. It had his name on it and his schedule for the day. "I got lost during that firefight."

"Oh right, now I remember you. Some animal name," the woman said. "Minx? Ferret?"

"Fox." Robert tossed the clipboard on the hammock and looked at them. "You're the married couple, right?"

Look like they are.

"Hell no, not married," the man said.

"We're in an open relationship," the woman said with a big wink at Robert. "I like that stubble you've grown, Mr. Liver."

"Jesus, Catherine, take it easy." To Robert he said, "Ms. Intestine here can't seem to tell the difference between a work environment and a bed."

"Sorry, but I'm already taken." Robert gave Catherine his best attempt at a leer. She had a great body, auburn hair parted in the middle, but a hard face with blood-hungry eyes. She smiled at him, and he was jolted to notice that one of her canines was long and fanglike. "I'm going to take a shower," he continued, noting the small bathroom with its door ajar behind them, "and no, Catherine, you can't join me."

She laughed like a goosed bear, and her partner just shook his head tiredly.

During all this, two other surgeons slept soundly in their hammocks.

Robert walked past Catherine on his way to the bathroom and she bumped her hip against him and said, "Hey, no need to be shy. You could undress out here. Show us what you got under there."

"Not happening." Robert hid a ripple of revulsion. "My mom raised me to be a nice southern gentleman."

"Nice?" came a deep voice from one of the hammocks. "Then what are you doing here, harvesting organs?"

Robert stopped and looked back at the hammocks. None of the sleepers seemed to have moved.

"Who said that?" he asked.

"Me." The answer came from the largest man in the room, his eyes still shut.

"He's the kidney guy," Catherine said, "and that's lung next to him. Kidney guy has quite the instrument, urologically speaking." Catherine's turtle eyes blinked slowly as she looked at Robert for his reaction.

"You're a piece of work, aren't you?" Robert said, trying to maintain what he remembered of Fox's southern drawl.

"Piece of something, anyway," came a higher pitched voice from the other hammock.

Lung.

Robert disappeared into the bathroom, glad to shut the door tightly behind him.

The shower was surprisingly strong, and he used the time to plot out his strategy. Ideally, he would recruit the surgeons against the narcos, but the surgeons seemed to be content hacking these innocent kids for their own profit.

They're just as guilty as the narcos, and they should pay for partaking in this organ harvesting—and for breaking medicine's golden rule: Primum non nocere.

First, do no harm.

Robert was on his own. He would have to be on guard and look for any opportunity to put these guys away.

And the narcos.

And rescue the kids …

Suddenly, the weight of the mission hit him.

Robert forced himself to shake off that last thought and got out of the shower, smelling slightly floral. In a cabinet he found a brand new pair of brown Dansko clogs and clean scrubs, which he donned gratefully, stuffing his filthy clothes in the large waste bin by the door.

When he re-entered the room, Catherine and her boyfriend were gone, the other two surgeons still lay corpselike in their hammocks, and on Robert's hammock someone had put a wrapped sandwich and a large, sealed bottle of water. He wolfed down the ham and cheese and chugged half the bottle before Graucho and another guard bustled into the room.

"Time," Graucho announced, and the surgeons moved out of their hammocks in one smooth motion.

"Fucking work," said the deep-voiced kidney man. "Worse than internship around here."

"Certainly better pay, though," the lung guy said, going for the hand sanitizer.

"No time to chat," the other guard shouted. He was a tall, skinny guy, his face screwed up like he had a mouthful of sore teeth. "Twenty kids to do. Another group tomorrow. Move. Let's go!"

The kidney doctor stopped dead, turned slowly, and walked right up to the hyped-up beanpole, who raised his gun and repeated, "Let's go!"

"We're moving fine," the big doctor said, his baritone seeming to wrap like a noose around the guard's neck. "Now you put that gun down or I'll shove it up your ass so far it'll give you another nose."

The guard turned and stepped out of the room with his back to the door, ignoring the big doctor and chanting, "Move it!"

Dr. Kidney stepped after him and pounded a fist between the twerp's shoulders, shutting him up but making him whirl and raise the gun again. Graucho quickly batted the gun aside and kicked the guard in the shins.

"Ouch!" he whined, stooping to rub it.

We're their moneymakers. Guards are here to protect us, not hurt us.

"Sorry, Dr. Massey," Graucho said. "We are on a tight schedule, but I'm sure you're aware of that. Whenever you're ready, we hope we can get started."

Massey snorted, got a gob of sanitizer in his meaty palm, started rubbing, and strolled out the door.

Followed by Lung.

Followed by Robert.

CHAPTER 30

The guards led them outside and across the square toward the second temple. Dr. Massey sang "Eye of the Tiger" with impressive bravura, and the twitchy guard turned around and scowled, which made him sing louder. Robert could see the crest of the hill where Guillermo hid, no doubt tracking their promenade through his binoculars. Robert quickly played his hand through his hair, sending finger code to him.

Action soon, thirty minutes.

Robert knew Guillermo would understand that meant he was going down into the cenotes, into the harvesting place, where he would attempt to put a stop to the whole operation. Robert reminded himself to keep an eye out for the directional arrows Guillermo had scored into the walls of the cenotes all those years ago.

They went into the temple, out of Guillermo's sightline. A somber quiet settled over Robert as the ancient walls seemed to heave a sigh of protest to this blasphemous intrusion. The sense of the past communicating to them sharpened when Robert realized that all four walls were filled with hieroglyphics: beautiful, ornate pictograms of brave citizens, earthly wonders, and scientific discoveries shining down from the stars.

Catherine's hyena laugh and the skinny guard's nasal bark jarred Robert back. Ahead of them was the entrance to a down staircase, located in the middle of the temple and flanked by two more guards. It was dimly lit by flickering light bulbs powered from a coughing generator. Robert was the last in the line and, as they started to descend, he wondered if now was the time to make his move. Although he had no weapons, he figured he could quickly kill the tired-looking guards at the entranceway, grab their rifles, mow down the others ahead of him, shoot the outside guards, and free the kids.

Too many to kill before they killed me, and Guillermo was expecting no action for a while yet.

Stick to the plan. See what's happening down below. There's stuff to put out of commission down there, and the tunnels below offer a better escape route.

But what about the kids outside?

Robert nodded pleasantly to the two guards at the entrance as he passed them. He hated being uncertain nearly as much as he hated this whole vile setup. It wasn't a peaceful feeling he carried down into the cenotes.

It was a writhing, throbbing, heart-pounding desire to rip limbs off bodies.

As they climbed down the many short steps, limestone grit crunched under their soles. The lights flickered and buzzed, the air grew cooler and damper. Finally they reached the bottom. It smelled of wet chalk. The space was a dark, dank enclosure with myriad stalactites like fingers pointing to a grave. On the floor, stalagmites created a series of paths. The group kept by the side of the small stream, which wound around and into the operating room.

The quiet gurgle of the stream mixed with the tinkling sounds of instruments being set out, equipment being prepared, and the dry human voices of the medical personnel already there. It was one of the eeriest scenes Robert had witnessed.

The evil and darkness contrasting to the natural beauty.

Robert spied a woman with a bottle of ketamine standing next to a man adjusting the knobs of an ophthalmoscope.

Our anesthesiologist and an ophthalmologist.

Two more heavily armed guards, looking more alert and competent than any Robert had seen yet, stood at the other end of the room. Their escort guards nodded at them and turned to go back the way they came.

To get the first patient.

Robert yawned as if bored, but really it was the awakening adrenaline surging into his blood vessels. He walked over to the equipment table and felt a queasy pang when he saw that it held every surgical device he would need for organ removal: retractors and pickups, scalpels, scissors, and a stack of different types of suture—nylon, Vicryl, Ethilon. Next to the table sat an ice machine and a bunch of coolers that would store the fresh-cut organs.

Next to the coolers sat a tall stack of huge leather-thick garbage bags.

For the remains of the victims.

"Okay," Massey boomed. "Might as well get this party started. Listen up. This is my third tour here, so I'm in charge. We'll leave the lungs and heart last so the other organs can stay oxygenated. Maybe you should start, Fox, with the liver. Then I'll do the kidneys. Catherine, you can take the pancreas, and then a breathtaking, heart-wrenching finish from the cardiopulmonary team. Joby, you can work on harvesting the corneas as soon as Fox starts the liver. Sound good?"

A few grunts of affirmation, and everybody began milling about in confused preparation.

No one likes being here. No one knows quite what to do.

Are they doing this against their will or just workers reluctant to put their nose to the grindstone?

"Here you are, Dr. Foxy."

Catherine had come up behind him and reached around his front holding out a sterile gown and surgical gloves, slowly grinding her pelvis and torso into his body. Robert snatched the gown and gloves and deftly stepped away from her.

Her smile in the flickering light looked like the start of a nightmare.

"Shouldn't we scrub before the surgery?" Robert asked.

Catherine raised an eyebrow. "Why?"

Robert paused.

My God.

Play it out.

"I'm just used to doing it, that's all," he said.

Her partner, the cardiovascular surgeon, had plunked himself down on the floor, where he leaned against the curved cave wall. His turn wouldn't be for a while. "Liver boy may have some nice brawn, Catherine, but I don't think he's got the brains of a laundry bag."

Massey had come over to give Robert a grizzly stare. "You afraid of infecting the patient? He's not going to have any organs after our surgeries, Fox. *Capiche*?"

"Sorry." Robert gulped. "Force of habit."

He could feel the gathering storm in him about to break.

The nearness of action calmed him.

"Okay," he said to Massey. "Back off. Let me do my thing."

"Spare us," Massey grunted and stepped away.

Robert took his time putting his gown on and slapped Catherine's hands away when she offered to help.

"Oh," she purred. "I love guys who play hard to get."

Robert shook his head. He gloved up, noting the positions of the two guards in the room, memorizing how they held their weapons.

And then he heard screaming that bunched his heart into a fist.

CHAPTER 31

Robert heard the shrill, high-pitched, grating sound of pure terror echoing through the walls of the cenotes.

Distant but piercing.

Approaching.

A young male was being dragged toward the operating room. The screams and howls never stopped; they got louder and more violent the closer they came.

"Jesus, punch the kid's lights out or let me dope him up," the anesthesiologist said. In appearance, she was a Norman Rockwell girl-next-door type, with apple cheeks and bright-yellow hair in a ponytail.

The two guards yanked in the teenage boy they had abused in the prison cage above. The long burn on his cheek was now a furious red. He fought with every ounce of energy he had, his adrenalized terror giving him twice his normal strength. The two operating room guards hurried to help restrain the prisoner, and soon all four got him strapped down on the operating table, though he still yelled and screamed.

"*Hijos de putas! Los voy a matar, cobardes de mierda!*"

The Barbie-doll anesthesiologist plunged a syringe in the boy's deltoid.

"Ketamine?" Robert asked.

She nodded and backed away. The boy started screaming again, and she put her hands over her ears, sat on a chair, and stared at the ground.

In the meantime, Robert glanced quickly around, evaluating every member of the team for potential allies.

He didn't seem to have any.

"What did you do to me?" the kid now yelled in broken English, changing his tune but not his volume as the drug swamped him. "Things are … spinning. *Que me pasa? Me … siento … mal …*"

His voice softened and his eyelids flickered like the lights strung above.

The anesthesiologist stood and went over to him and took his pulse, biting her lip.

The boy's eyes suddenly sprang open, and he growled at her in a voice deeper than Massey's. "*Kinach'ayo uwach ulew!*"

Then he went unconscious.

A lava-hot ripple ran up Robert's spine.

The anesthesiologist looked utterly shocked and dropped the boy's wrist, putting her hand to her mouth and staring at him in awe. "What the hell is 'Kinach'ayo uwach ulew?'"

"It's nonsense," Catherine said, shaking her head.

"Actually, it was old Mayan," Robert said, without thinking. He had recognized the language and phrase from his days of Mayan obsession.

"Sure it was," the cardiovascular surgeon scoffed.

"No, it was." Robert adjusted his surgical gloves. "I did a big Mayan language thing for a college elective. One of the reasons I signed up for this work—I wanted to see the temples."

"As well as make the big bucks, of course," said the ophthalmologist, a gnome-like man with what looked like a rash of warts on the back of both hands.

Robert sighed internally, realizing now that Guillermo wasn't completely nuts for wanting to kill Fox when they'd found him.

"What he screamed roughly translates to"—Robert gave the shaken anesthesiologist a soft look—"We are all children of the sun."

"Whatever," she mumbled and proceeded to attach the kid to the breathing apparatus.

Then there was silence, except for her grunt-tinged efforts and the mechanical indifference of the machine noises. Robert took a quick scan around and could see bitterness and distaste etched into every slack-jawed face.

Finished, the anesthesiologist plopped into a chair. "Let's get this over with."

One of the two guards who had escorted the boy said to Massey, "We're supposed to bring the next one down. How long before you get going?"

"Go get him," Massey said irritably, seeming to snap awake. "And knock that one out before you bring him down here. All the screaming is giving me a headache. We're supposed to be down here for the next twelve hours."

"Okay," the guard said, then spat and left with his partner.

Two down, two to go.

"Come on, Fox, get to it," Massey said. "Make the incision, get the liver, and get out of the way."

Robert stared at the unconscious kid lying before him.

Now what?

He looked around. The two guards were screwing silencers on their revolvers.

"Cold feet?" One of them pointed the gun at Robert with a steady hand.

Robert laughed, feeling his fight-or-flight energy cranking to the fight side. "Not at all," he said. "I just don't think we should do this guy first."

All six physicians turned to Robert with raised eyebrows.

"Excuse me?" Massey said, moving toward Robert like a goaded bully.

"Look at the pallor on the kid," Robert said, sounding confident. "I've had more experience with extraction than you all put together. Take my word for it. His organs are not going to be fit. They would pollute all the others. He's anemic."

In fact, the boy's coffee skin was milky, his recent traumas having no doubt paled him with fright.

"That's bullshit," the cardiovascular surgeon said. "It's not up to you to decide whether we harvest or not. And who gives a fuck about the condition of the organs? They'll sell them anyway, and the buyers will keep coming and shelling out. Can we just get on with it, for Christ's sake? Get it done and maybe have time left for some partying tonight?"

"Goddamn it, Fox, if you won't make the first incision, I will." Massey tried to shoulder Robert aside.

Robert held his ground with resilience and sheer body strength—which seemed to startle Massey, who was used to throwing his weight around.

"Cool it," Robert said, the steel in his voice prodding Massey back a step. Robert bent and pulled the boy's eyelids down. "Look at this. Pale conjunctiva. And the skin … Did you guys go to medical school? Can't you diagnose pallor? What the fuck do you think this is, albinism? You guys don't have a clue what malnourishment can do to these kids. You want to start this whole barrel of surgeries off with a rotten apple? You don't think that's going to cut into our fee base in the long run? The receiving surgeons are bound to notice the poor quality of the organs. Let's be smart about this, okay? Put this kid over in a corner somewhere and let's wait for the next one."

"What are you doing?" Massey snapped, as if suddenly coming awake. "That's not anemia!"

Shit.

"If it isn't," Robert snapped right back, "it's something worse!"

"We should listen to Fox," the general surgeon said.

"Who gives a shit, Catherine?" Massey barked. "Let's just get this done. If you or Fox don't want to, get the hell out of here."

"No one's leaving," came the guard's voice from behind, and Robert felt the silencer gently tap-tap-tap on his head.

Robert turned. It was the guard with the steady hand, who now had backed a safe distance away but kept the gun aimed coolly at Robert's third eye.

No jumping this guy.

His eyes met the guard's and Robert felt a warrior recognition pass between them.

The guard moved back two more feet, his hand never wavering.

Robert smiled.

The guard smiled back. "So whose blood are we going to see next, doc? Yours or the kid's?"

Robert's chest was threatening to explode. He turned and picked up the scalpel and calculated the chances of whirling and heaving it through the guard's eye before his gun went off, but then the other guard stepped in front of Robert, gun raised.

"All right, everyone," Robert said. "Could we all relax a bit? Why so touchy? You gun guys … back off, please. Give me some room to breathe."

The guards backed away and took up their former positions, their guns still leveled at Robert.

"Okay," Robert said, defeated. He looked around at the other physicians. "I'll start."

"Just cut, asshole." Massey turned to the anesthesiologist. "Henrietta, start the kid on propofol and intubate him."

"Just remember." Robert raised his scalpel. "I thought this was a bad idea. We shouldn't be using hypoxic organs from an anemic patient."

"For ten thousand per organ, I don't give a fuck if the kid's anemic." Henrietta pushed the milky-white medication through a newly inserted IV and got the respirator, the Miller blade, and the 6-0 tube ready for intubation.

As Robert made the incision along the boy's upper right quadrant, his mind sped through a rationalization of his actions.

Sacrifice.

The boy's death will save the lives of thousands of others.

I'm not killing him, I'm just taking his liver. The others will be the murderers. When they start harvesting, I can go after the guards.

I have no other choice.

The boy's bright red blood seeped through the incision, and Robert prayed he'd be able to live with himself once this all played out.

CHAPTER 32

Robert always prided himself on having the steadiest hands. It was a matter of breathing. No matter how difficult, pressured, or anxious he was, awareness of his breath guided him with grace through anything—whether shooting a gun or an arrow, harnessing his rage, taming a panic, or finding the flow when he had to perform an emergency procedure.

As he continued the incision through the subcutaneous tissue and fascia, he used his breathing to slow his thumping heart and keep his racing mind from distracting him. His thoughts distilled down to one.

If I take out his liver and attack them after, will this kid survive?

Robert needed to believe the boy would.

"All right, I'm visualizing the liver now," he said.

"Good," Massey said. "Don't take forever. I'll start prepping for the kidneys."

"Don't bother." Robert pointed to the liver. "The boy has Gaucher's disease."

"Gaucher's?" Massey came over and peered into the cavity.

"I told you, goddamn it!" Robert snapped. "Look at that hepatomegaly. The spleen's enlarged, too. The kid has an inborn error of metabolism affecting his liver. If I take it out, it'll turn necrotic in about an hour, and so will all the other organs. I told you to listen to me. Jesus Christ! You guys think hauling up a box of necrotic organs to start the show will make us look good? Head guy is going to have our necks. He'll kill us all and get himself another set of surgeons to do his harvesting."

The doctors exchanged wary glances.

Then Massey spoke in a grave voice, distractedly massaging the shoulder he had bumped against Robert earlier. "Necrotic is no good. No good at all. I'm not going down for that. Fox is right. He's an obnoxious prick, maybe, but he's right. Fernando!" He called to the second-best guard. "Go tell them to hustle the next one up."

Fernando scuttled out.

Robert exhaled in relief under his mask and started to close the patient up.

"What are you doing, Fox?" the warty ophthalmologist snorted. "Get out of that kid already. Let Henrietta pull his breathing tube out and let him bleed out."

"Not chancing him infecting anything." Robert tightened the stitches.

Henrietta lifted her head up. "Do you want me to extubate him?"

"In a sec." Robert was in the zone with his stitching, and Massey came over to watch.

"The prick can tie," Massey said. "You got great hands, Fox!"

Robert breathed deep and steady. His stitching went on in a hitchless blur. Massey's sounds of approval even drew Henrietta out of her chair to come watch.

Robert finished the last stitch and pulled back, wiping the sweat from his brow. Catherine clapped a few times while Henrietta unhooked the kid from the breathing machine.

While mopping his brow, Robert noticed the one remaining guard briefly rub his eyes.

As Henrietta finished taking out the breathing tube, Robert put the retractors and leftover suture back on the instrument table and palmed two scalpels.

Then he heard the screeching of a young woman being brought toward the operating room.

Now or never.

The steadiness of his breathing while operating now served to keep his combat movements sure and strong. He pivoted and threw a scalpel into the guard's left eye, instantly sending the man's brain into spasms. The doctors gasped and yelled as the guard crumpled to the floor. Instantly Robert had the dying guard's silencered gun in his own hand and turned it on all the doctors.

"All you maggots, bunch together behind Massey there! No warning shouts and I'll spare your lives."

From the entry tunnel came the sound of two awful blows, and the girl's screams turned to an extended hoarse croaking with a ghastly echo. Massey spoke in a panicky whisper to Robert. "Have you gone crazy, man?"

The girl's croaking now turned to a loud retching.

A shaky young voice floated up from the operating table. "Rosa? Is that you, *hermana?*"

The boy was waking up already.

"You're all murderers," Robert hissed. "I should shoot you all."

The three guards and the pain-racked girl were just yards away from the entryway now, and Henrietta tried to yell a warning.

With the precision of a surgeon, Robert embedded a scalpel in the middle of her larynx, silencing her.

Forever.

"Guards!" Massy yelled.

Robert's silencered gun splattered the speech center in the big guy's brain all over the doctors behind him.

"What's going on?" Fernando asked the guard, stepping back into the operating arena. His eyes widened at the gore in the flickering lights, and Robert shot him precisely where the spine meets the brainstem.

Instant death.

Without pause Robert walked out into the tunnel, firing multiple shots and killing the other two guards.

He walked back in the operating room with a ten-year-old girl clinging to his side, doubled over in pain and panting.

"Rosa?"

The boy had managed to undo one of his straps and was raising himself up.

"Mateo!" his sister cried and ran to him, tearing at his straps.

Soon the boy was free. He sat up slowly, looking dazed.

Robert stood in place breathing deeply and evenly.

Calculating.

He felt like Thor calling forth the serpent.

CHAPTER 33

The general surgeon, the pulmonologist, the cardiovascular surgeon, and the ophthalmologist seemed too stunned by the violence to be any threat. Robert quickly undid his scrubs and began to remove the dead guard's uniform. The brother and sister were rallying, taking strength from each other.

"Get yourselves ready," Robert said to them as he began donning the guard's uniform. "I'm getting you out of this hellhole."

"Let me help." Catherine snatched up Robert's scrubs and angrily wiped Massey's brain gore off her scrub top. "I'm ashamed I was involved in all of this. I never wanted to do it in the first place. My boyfriend dragged me into it."

"I did not," the cardiovascular surgeon shot back.

"Please," Catherine urged, her eyes welling up. "Let me make amends for what I've done."

Buttoning up the guard's uniform, Robert cast his fiercest diagnostic eye over her.

Tears in her eyes—shame and grief seemed real.

Shoulders back defiantly, slumping gone, seeming determined—also real.

"Okay, Catherine," he said.

"Cathy," she snapped, all business, knowing time was short.

"Whatever." He put the guard's cap on, pleased with its fit. "Put the rest of these scumbags out. Use ketamine."

The three remaining doctors were too shaken to object.

"Give me your cell," Robert said.

Without missing a beat, she slipped it from her back pocket and tossed it to him. He used it to take their pictures, telling them, "You are all going down. I got your pictures, and I'll get your names. You'll never see the inside of an operating room again. I'll be coming back for you someday, believe me. You're all co-conspirators for attempted murder, and Cathy might be going to prison with you, depending on how she does now."

Cathy plunged the needle into her boyfriend, who didn't fight her. He went unconscious with the rest of them in seconds.

Mateo was now trying to walk, making involuntary sounds of pain. "Cathy, fix him up with something. Draw up twenty micrograms of Fentanyl and give him a shot. We have to get moving!"

"Got it." She pulled a syringe of fentanyl and gave Mateo just enough to ease his pain, but not enough to prevent him from walking.

"Tough it out, Mateo." Robert grabbed the boy's arm and helped him walk to the doorway. "The medication will kick in soon."

"*Estoy bien,*" the kid said, gritting his teeth. "Where are we going?"

"One sec," Robert said. "Cathy, hold him up."

Cathy was holding the young girl's hand, and with her free arm she steadied Mateo. Robert stepped into the passageway. The two guards lay on the bloody limestone floor, one with his blasted head getting sluiced by the small stream. Robert collected their weapons and ammunition and a small flashlight. He paused and listened intently for any sound of approaching trouble.

"Let's go," he called back in a loud whisper. The three came out and made their way to Robert. As she looked at the corpses, the girl let out a snarl of hate.

"Shh, *relajate.*" Robert put a gentle hand on her shoulder.

Cathy bent her face down to the girl's. "Okay, Rosa. Quiet as you can now. We don't want anyone hearing us, okay?"

Rosa lurched forward and violently kicked the torso of one of the guards and spat on the other's decimated head. Then she and her brother shared a smile. "*Vamos.*" She nodded to the shocked Cathy.

Robert used the flashlight to examine the cave walls. "Everyone! Come over here."

They scuttled over to look. A gouged out symbol appeared in the middle of the limestone wall: an arrow pointing forward.

The work of an ingenious, brave orphan from years ago.

"These arrows lead you from here into the woods," he whispered. "You'll probably find them wherever the tunnels branch. My friend Guillermo should be outside to meet you. Trust him with your life. And Cathy—you have to always tell him the truth. He's a bloodhound for lies."

"Aren't you coming with us?" Cathy asked, slightly panicked.

"I have to free the rest of the kids first."

They went without incident to the stairs leading up to the temple, where three tunnels branched. Sure enough, a rough-hewn arrow pointed the way. By now, Mateo was moving with stronger legs, bent over slightly with a hand covering his stitches. Robert stood by the arrow and checked the staircase for anyone descending. Cathy and the kids passed and went around a bend ahead. Robert started to follow, but he heard a rough male voice coming from ahead.

"Stop right there!"

Another guard.

"I'm one of the doctors," he heard Cathy say in a strong voice.

"You're going the wrong way," the guard growled.

Robert quietly placed his guns on the ground and took out the hunting knife he had taken from one of the dead guards.

"Hola!" he yelled and then quickly stepped into sight of the guard saying, "Ah, there you are. Amigo! I'm Doctor Fox. We made a wrong turn by the staircase."

"Why are you wearing those clothes?" the guard asked.

"Graucho gave them to me," Robert said, shrugging. "I got blood on my scrubs during the last surgery."

"What are you doing with the product?" The guard pointed the gun barrel at the glaring children.

"Shh," Cathy said, conspiratorially. "You know what we do with the product but they don't, so let's keep them calm, comprende?"

Just then the guard's walkie-talkie crackled with static and an urgent voice blared out in Spanish: "All units to the operating room! Secure a man there called Dr. Fox. He's an imposter and dangerous."

"*Joder!*" the guard cursed and swung the barrel at Robert, pulling the trigger.

"No!" Cathy yelled as she jumped at the barrel. The shot took the top left chunk of her auburn head off, deflecting the bullet that passed Robert so closely he heard its Doppler buzz.

Before he knew what he had done, he had rammed the knife blade sideways into the guard's ear, stepped around the gaping kids, and broken the guard's neck with one savage twist.

"Cathy!" Robert called, kneeling down. She was now on her back, panting hoarsely, her eyes seeing faraway horrors.

Her eyes swam back into focus, recognizing Robert.

"So … sorry," she gurgled.

"I can carry you." Robert put his hands under her shoulders.

A look of surprise came over her.

Then Robert recognized the clayish appearance of a body abandoned by whatever once had animated it.

CHAPTER 34

"*Vayan*," Robert said to the kids, giving Rosa the flashlight. "Look for the arrows."

"Gracias," they both said and trudged ahead, quickly disappearing from sight.

Robert grabbed the guard's walkie-talkie and the two grenades on his utility belt. He took the guard's thick black glasses, pushed the lenses out, and donned them for disguise. Then he backtracked, picked up the weapons he had put on the floor, and made his way back to the staircase.

How the hell did they find out I wasn't Fox?

His uniform and glasses might hide him for a while, but they were on the lookout for him.

He heard several sets of running footsteps converging on the staircase and pulled the guard's hat further down on his forehead. Then he began to run, as if he were also a guard called to the operating room to take hold of the duplicitous Dr. Fox.

As he neared the staircase, he saw four guards stomping down it and two others emerging from different tunnel branches.

They all met at the bottom of the stairs and huddled. Robert came up behind them, drawing no particular notice, hearing hushed orders to barge into the OR without hurting "the product."

They ran ahead, but Robert stayed. Ten yards away they stopped and as one turned back to him.

"*Vamos!*" one ordered in Spanish.

"Catch!" Robert yelled back, lobbing two grenades at them and scampering up the stairs three at a time.

The double explosion beneath was followed by despairing cries.

"A gift from karma," Robert snarled under his breath and emerged into the temple area.

Four more guards.

Two at the entrance, two trotting toward him with worried looks.

"*Todo bien,*" Robert shouted at them, waving them back. "Just a tank of chloroform overheated."

"*Que?*" called one of the entrance guards.

"Who the hell are you?" asked one of the approaching guards, who looked like an adolescent.

"They told me to get a machine gun," Robert shouted at him with great urgency, grabbing the barrel of the Uzi the guard had raised at him.

"No!" the startled guard yelled. "What are you doing ..."

Robert raised his other arm with the AK-47 and blasted the two near guards, wrestling the Uzi away as they fell and deftly turned it on the guards at the entrance. He mowed them down with a three-second spray.

He scuttled to the entrance and peered out. A line of guards rushed toward the machine gun sounds. He rapidly shot the legs from under eight of them, and then skeet-shot a grenade coming toward him in the air and ducked.

Flying shrapnel from the detonated grenade wounded two more.

Robert sprinted toward the cage filled with excited, shouting prisoners, but then stopped dead as fire from above splintered the wooden walkway ahead of him.

The guards in the tower.

He skittered back into the temple. Their vantage point was too commanding.

Then he heard a distant shot, a descending scream, and the body of one of the tower guards landing with a thud three feet from Robert.

Guillermo!

Robert positioned himself in the entranceway so Guillermo could spot him, and hand-signaled: *two prisoners coming to you.*

A mirror flashed a light code to Robert.

Message received.

A guard unexpectedly jumped on Robert's back and he fell forward. A powerful forearm pressed against his throat. Robert reached up and jabbed two fingers in his assailant's eye. The forearm released as the guard let out a high-pitched girlish whine, and Robert twisted around to see his attacker.

Baraka.

Still sobbing, Baraka tried to yank a pearl-handled revolver from his shoulder holster.

Robert heard a gunshot from a distance, then smiled as he noted Baraka looking at the distant horizon, as if trying to see the hole that had bloomed in his forehead.

He fell down.

Dead.

Robert whirled around to find Guillermo in the unseen distance. A light winked.

Under cover of fire, a swarm of guards approached.

And still one guard on top of the temple.

Guillermo's high-powered weaponry started raining blasts on the guards, but they had scoped his position out and were keeping out of his sightline.

These guards will get to me before I can get to the kids.

Guillermo will have to deal with freeing the prisoners.

Robert turned and ran down the staircase, into the cenotes. He wasn't sure what his plan was now. The primary rule of battle was taking over.

Survive.

Live to fight another hour.

Maybe the cenotes had other staircases or tunnels up to the compound.

Robert ran as the contingencies sped through his military brain.

Can't go to the operating room—too many soldiers were ordered there.

He passed the eight soldiers he had blasted into death. Three remained alive, one groaning. Without compunction, he ran past them. Cathy's cell gave off a fine bright flashlight glow.

The sound of military boots tramped in even cadence.

A great number of boots.

Robert came to the three branching tunnels by the staircase and zoomed down a tunnel not taken before, the cell light showing the way.

Running for his life.

It seemed that no matter where he ran the sound of approaching guards got louder.

Surrounding me? How would they know?

Does the walkie-talkie have a GPS?

Running full speed, he looked at the two-way radio. No GPS or any modern feature—just the plain old clunky hand-held he remembered from battles twenty years ago, fighting guerillas with Guillermo.

They are flooding the tunnels with guards, trying to surround me.

The corridor started to slope up. Dim light filtered through the ceiling; it gave the area an eerie glow, shadowed weirdly by the hanging stalactites.

As Robert ran, he noticed that the stalactites became longer and heavier, and the light filtering down grew brighter.

And the soldiers came closer and closer.

Without slowing down he veered and ran up the wall, falling off toward a hanging stalactite after three steps. He kept his legs in motion to gain leverage against the structures, slanting himself further upward. Finally, he touched the ceiling with his belly, wrapped his legs around the base of a curved stalactite, then caught the backs of his knees over its swoosh-shaped hook.

Hanging there like a bat.

Letting his breath even out.

Hearing boots splashing through the small stream around the bend, Robert carefully unstrapped the Uzi from his shoulder and waited.

CHAPTER 35

Six guards rushed through the narrow limestone corridor. Robert slaughtered each one.

The smoke and stench of the gunfire filled the area, mingling with the rusty smell of blood.

Battle incense for the warrior reloading above.

More will come to the sounds of carnage.

More came, peering everywhere in dazed fear.

Everywhere but up.

Robert rained down bullets like a storm of molten hail.

Two guards managed to shoot up at Robert before falling, their bullets slamming holes in the thin ceiling.

A broad shaft of light fell on Robert.

Squinting, he righted himself and clambered up into the day, onto a patch of earth on the periphery of the Kundal ruins.

A yard away were two dead guards wearing the same uniform as Robert. He belly-crawled over and played dead beside them, assessing the situation.

He heard commotion and shouts from various areas, but no shots or explosions.

Why had Guillermo stopped firing?

Without thinking, he craned his neck for a better view and saw the makeshift prison, manned by three guards.

Robert heard a *pop* and felt a bullet scratch his cheek. He wiped at it, and his hand came back bloody.

Another bullet thunked wetly into the corpse of the guard beside him, jolting Robert up into a furious zig-zag sprint toward the prison, readying his AK-47 to fire when there was no danger of hitting the prisoners. The Uzi thumped painfully against his back as he ran, but he felt no pain. Bullets sprayed around him but something in his finely tuned and now highly revved warrior's body guided him flawlessly. He was doing a beautiful gliding survival dance to the mad drumming of the gunfire and his booming heart.

He saw his window for a safe series of shots at the cage guards, who now saw him coming and were raising their weapons.

Robert sent off another wave of bullets.

The guards went down but Robert sensed others coming sideways at him, so he swerved and took refuge behind a limestone Mayan statue.

As he crouched there panting, his walkie-talkie suddenly crackled and a rich baritone voice boomed out, echoed by other walkie-talkies spread throughout the compound.

"Dr. McKenzie." The voice gave Robert a full-body shudder. "Stop and look at the top of the temple."

Robert looked up.

He saw a sight that momentarily overshadowed all the other atrocities he'd seen so far that day: his friend Guillermo, tied and hanging from a rafter, his toes resting on a seventy-five–foot high temple platform, motionless.

Without another thought, Robert aimed at the guard standing next to Guillermo.

But then something sharp hit the back of his head.

And everything turned black.

CHAPTER 36

Robert's eyelids cracked open and flickered at the burning sunlight. When they steadied enough, he realized the courtyard was far below, and his first thought was that he was flying.

He had turned into a spirit falcon to escape all the gunfire and was soaring up to Guillermo's rescue.

Then an electric pain knifed down his arms and cleared the dreams from his mind. His red-misted vision settled on the rope digging into his wrists.

He was on a platform seventy-five feet in the air, tied by his wrists to a rafter on the mount of the Mayan high temple. Guillermo dangled across from him, also bound, head hanging, bleeding from his mouth and ears.

Dead?

Guillermo's chest heaved and a faint ragged groan escaped his mouth.

Alive.

A drop of blood abruptly smeared Robert's eyes, turning everything deeper red. He shook his head to clear his vision and began assessing his wounds.

Scalp laceration: superficial. Neurological deficits: absent. Therefore, no intracranial bleed or cerebral contusion.

He rotated his head a bit.

Supple neck, no midline pain.

No cervical spinal fractures.

A series of buzzing pains did a brief drill up and down his arms, making him gasp.

Arms sore from hanging but no major trauma. Ribs throbbing—beaten or kicked when I was unconscious.

He took a deep breath, and little lightning bolts shot across his ribs.

Contusions along ribs six and seven bilaterally. Possibly fractured. Lungs fine, not collapsed or filling with blood. No shortness of breath or dyspnea.

Therefore, no pneumothorax or hemothorax.

Legs? Fine, good movement.

All things considered, stable.

Then a blow to his sternum changed his mind, followed by a rifle butt into his sore ribs.

As he struggled to regain his breath, Robert felt a series of slaps to his face. When he opened his eyes, Robert observed that the young guard beating him was staring into his eyes with an almost inhuman curiosity, waiting for Robert to revive enough so he could beat him into semiconsciousness again.

"I'm going to kill you," Robert yelled, receiving three mechanically precise flank punches in response.

"I hardly think you're in a position to make threats, *cabron*. And I wouldn't try your luck with Angelo," came a voice behind him. "Angelo, in fact, we call him Diablo. He's very interested in how to make you suffer as much as possible without passing out. He's become quite the expert under my instructions about anatomy and the human pain response."

"Who's talking?" Robert rasped. "Show yourself!"

Diablo raised his rifle butt again and prepared for another blow.

"Enough, Diablo!"

At this command the guard bowed and backed away, and a thin man in an immaculate uniform appeared in front of Robert. Intelligence radiated from his face, as well as something deeply twisted from his eyes.

"I suggest you start behaving yourself, Dr. McKenzie," the man said. "We're taking it easy on you for now. Don't test our patience."

"Who the hell are you?" Robert needed to keep the man speaking until he could better assess his situation. He needed to figure out a way to save Guillermo and escape. "I see you more clearly now, and my opinion hasn't changed. I'm going to kill both of you."

"Enough of your bravado, Dr. McKenzie. Any more from your mouth, I'll simply take a minute and cut your tongue out."

"How do you know my name?"

"I'll ask the questions," the man yelled, the keenness of his exasperation making Robert blink. "Who do you think you are, messing up my operation here to provide organs for needy people everywhere? Has this old man corrupted your medical objectivity so completely?"

"I know that voice," Guillermo whispered without looking up.

"Do you?" The man whirled and stuck his face into Guillermo's.

"Joaquin," Guillermo muttered, opening his eyes wide and steady, startling the man.

"I'm impressed you remember me."

"This is Joaquin?" Robert asked. "This unhinged psycho is the good brother of the trio?"

"Psycho?" Joaquin shrieked. "Does this empire I've set up here look like the work of a *psycho*?"

As the beady-eyed guard watched Joaquin pace and steam, Robert tried to work his wrists out of his ropes—but they were far too tight. From the corner of his eye, he caught a signal from Guillermo.

Leg scissors when we both have a shot.

Robert nodded, just as Joaquin turned and walked aggressively at Guillermo, pulled his head up, and studied the multiple bruises on his face.

"Colorful," he said with satisfaction, then nodded to the guard at his shoulder. "Pretty work."

The guard beamed, and the duo came over to Robert.

"No doubt, Dr. McKenzie, like any sophomoric liberal," Joaquin began in what seemed like a calm, reasonable tone, "you are unable to see the visionary reach of my operation here. Unable to fathom the superior good it does. Only able to harp at its minor drawbacks."

"You're crazy," Robert said.

"As I suspected," Joaquin said. "A mind drenched in *vin ordinaire*."

Guillermo spoke up softly. "You think organs do greater good in rich people than in poor people. That's what you call *visionary*?"

"Ah," Joaquin said, "my old teacher, still a bleeding heart."

"Eviscerated Guatemalan kids are more than minor drawbacks," Robert said.

"Ever hear of Nietzsche?" Joaquin laughed. "I'm simply his disciple. I'm his *Übermensch*. I don't need organized religion to tell me to do good so I can enjoy an afterlife. *This* is my afterlife, and I'm Nietzsche's superman."

"I taught you how to heal," came Guillermo's pleading voice. "Remember the vow you swore to me before you left for medical school?"

"Don't waste your breath," Joaquin snapped. A guilty panic flitted across his face. "I've gone beyond your sentimental bullshit!"

"Joaquin," Guillermo whispered. "Don't do this. It's never too late to quit doing harm. Remember what your father said before he died."

"What did he say?" Joaquin asked.

"He …" Guillermo whispered, but so softly he knew Joaquin couldn't quite hear him.

"What are you saying about my father?" Joaquin barked. He moved closer to Guillermo. Diablo moved with him but stopped when Robert hissed, "Diablo."

As Diablo turned back with an irritated frown, Guillermo said to Joaquin, "Your father …"

"My father what?" Joaquin said menacingly, getting in Guillermo's face.

"Your father … loved you!" Guillermo yelled and jackknifed up. So did Robert, and in seconds their criss-crossed legs were choking the life from their captors. With a sudden heave, Robert slung the gurgling Diablo over the side of the high platform and his falling scream of terror mixed with Joaquin's grunts as he tried to free himself and catch a lungful of oxygen.

"Ready here!" Robert called out.

With a burst of energy, Guillermo levered Joaquin toward Robert, who launched a vicious kick directly into Joaquin's gasping face. The kick broke Joaquin's nose, but didn't knock him down. With a howl, he spun around, both hands over his face.

Robert and Guillermo were now both swinging and spinning from their tied wrists. Robert aimed another kick, and the tip of his boot smacked into Joaquin's groin. As

Joaquin grabbed at his groin, Guillermo swung his foot for a knockout uppercut.

But Joaquin saw it coming and backed away just as the would-be-fatal blow swooshed harmlessly past his nose.

Joaquin was now aware enough to keep his body out of reach from his captives.

Game over.

Robert panted, seething. He looked at Guillermo, and a signal passed between them that had never been prearranged.

Lost that round.

Robert nodded. Guillermo grimaced.

They were in for it.

CHAPTER 37

Joaquin straightened up slowly, shaking his head, a death's-head smile twisting his face. He wiped blood from his nose with his sleeve, rattled a command into his walkie-talkie, tucked the device back in his belt, and looked back and forth between Robert and Guillermo with something like amused admiration.

"I should have known to be more careful. I should've hog-tied you before stringing you up."

"You're some superman," Robert said. "You got a busted nose and a couple of sore nuts."

"Just a scratch." Joaquin tilted his nose skyward. "Someone is coming to pay back with interest the pain you've given me."

"You kill children," Robert said. "You rip their hearts out. Their blood screams at you every minute."

"How pretty for you to think so," Joaquin said, now fully plastered with that unearthly calm he used to deaden his eyes. "Like all great men, I carry an immense sorrow as I wade through red streams toward the clear light of a new day. Like Napoleon, like Che, like the Contras, like Bush and Cheney. It takes blood to give life to the new world body. Terribly sad, in a way, but absolutely necessary if life is to evolve."

"You're going to pay for this," Guillermo said, and this drew Joaquin's distant stare back into local focus.

"Don't threaten me, old man."

"Your father was my best friend," Guillermo said. "I brought you into this world."

"And I thank you for that," Joaquin said. "My father was your friend, right? So why when I was four did my father, your best friend, die in Guatemala City like a dog?" Joaquin's voice rose to a hysterical pitch. "He could've lived. No one thought to treat his hyperkalemia? Your great medical know-how didn't get anyone there to give him hemodialysis? He had to die like a rabid dog from something that could've been treated by either dialysis or … Guess what? A goddamn kidney transplant! That's right. One simple organ from even the stupidest, most useless dolt in the Guatemalan jungles. You might not have learned anything from the death of someone you called a friend, but my father's death put a purpose in me."

"You can't be serious." Guillermo's head hung with pain and fatigue. "You can't really believe your father is smiling as your men drag a screaming girl onto an operating table and vivisect her. You're disgracing his memory."

"His memory? I don't need to remember him. He's alive now. I can sense his presence in all my thoughts. Great men are free from low-grade compunctions that keep us bound to this dull earth. We see in terms of eons, in terms of seismic shifts in consciousness. The truth was right before my eyes when my father died, and he had to die for me to see it. Our great Guatemalan jungle has the key to a higher class of humanity: an endless supply of trouble-free organs. Less hassle from authority. Less paperwork. Less bribery. More life for those with the money and power to improve quality of life."

Robert racked his brain trying to think of any way he could get through Joaquin's craziness. He didn't mind letting him rant on: the longer he talked, the longer Robert and Guillermo avoided torture.

"Economics is the real grace heaven sends us," Joaquin went on. "Selling some girl to the sex trade will get me no more than ten thousand dollars. But selling her organs? Do the math." He paused and smiled. "Her kidney? Two hundred thousand. Her heart, lungs, and liver? A cool half million each. And if I really want to be noble, I can also harvest the corneas, skin—even her ovaries. Did you know they've started transplanting ovaries? It's amazing what modern medicine can do. And we're on the cutting edge."

"Of course." Robert tried to buy some time. "The drug trade is old world. Now getting even more outmoded thanks to the legalization of marijuana in the U.S."

"Exactly! But organs? Tell me, Dr. McKenzie. How many people die waiting for a transplant?"

"I have no idea." Robert focused. If Joaquin came a foot closer he'd be within his reach again.

"I'll tell you. Twenty people a *day*!" Joaquin shook his head. "Ridiculous, given the abundance of robust organs we have here in our resource-rich rainforest. Poor people all over this place. People not worth the pits they piss in. Most of them will end up dying anyway of some tropical disease. You know that, right? Eight million kids die before their eighth birthday in the developing world. A sad fact for some, an exciting revelation for my partners and I."

"You vowed as a doctor," came Guillermo's weakening voice, "to preserve life, to save *all* life. *Primum non nocere.* First do no harm, remember? All people are equal in the eyes of God—and physicians."

"But I do save life," Joaquin shot back, looking elated to reverse the teacher-student role with his old mentor. "A single one of these filthy villagers can save eight well-dressed, bright-minded citizens of the world. Think about it—you haven't forgotten how to count, have you? Two kidneys, two lungs, a heart, and a liver partitioned into three. It's just as our brilliant prophet Machiavelli declared: The end justifies the means."

The quote made Robert think so piercingly of his discussions with Sharon that he almost vomited. The fear of not seeing her again obliterated Joaquin's drivel. When he finally willed his awareness back into the moment, he heard Joaquin still carrying on.

"Do you know how much a rich parent would pay for an organ for their promising young child?"

"You just told us. Black market price for a kidney is two hundred thousand," Robert said.

"That's right, Dr. McKenzie. But for a rich parent in Beverly Hills with a child with polycystic kidney disease? They've paid a million for a single kidney, and they usually prefer the matched set. That's two million. And a heart and lung transplant? I had a parent of a child with Tetralogy of Fallot pay me five million. The father was, in fact, a heartless investment banker. The best kind. He didn't balk at forking over the money, and now his kid is getting an MBA from Stanford." Joaquin paused for a moment. "Livers are the new gold mine. All the more precious because newborns tend to die so quickly of inborn errors of metabolism. So sad, but so glorious! Get in touch with a weepy, filthy-rich parent through hospital connections—*ka-ching*!"

Robert heard a roar overhead.

"Ah, that's my ride," Joaquin said. "The new guard should be a pleasant surprise for you. I think I hear him coming up now." He called down the stairs and waved, then turned back to Robert and Guillermo. "Gentlemen, it's been great fun showing you the light and having you tickle my nose and balls. But now I'm off to Guatemala City to gather more men and surgeons." He was shouting now, to be heard over the roar of the helicopter landing in the square below. He stretched out his hand to help the arriving guard onto the platform. "I believe you all know each other, so I'll leave you in capable hands. Adios!"

With a wave, Joaquin disappeared down the stairs.

Leaving the new guard staring at them, the rotor wind blowing his hair, the look in his eyes pure malice.

Dr. Fox.

Holding a baseball bat.

CHAPTER 38

"I guess this explains how they figured out I wasn't you," Robert said.

"It does," Fox drawled, taking some short, lazy swings with the aluminum bat.

"I bet I know how you got away." Guillermo no longer sounded tired. "You had a GPS in your shoe? That big heel, made you look taller than the punk you are?"

"You should be nice, old man." Fox stepped toward Guillermo, ready to bat him one.

"Hey!" Robert yelled.

Fox turned with bemusement.

"Is that true about the GPS? Did your buddies sneak you out of our village?"

"It was a little more than that. Not only did I escape your tick-infested little swamp of huts," Fox said, "I also had the pleasure of seeing it burned to the ground, brown-skinned bodies all over the place like night crawlers after a rain. And my favorite good time was pounding the gourd-head on one Dr. Mel, your late friend, into pumpkin relish. If you're worried if he suffered much, I can only say … yeah, he did. Judging, that is, from the endless pig-squeals."

"You son of a bitch!" Robert cried.

Fox stepped forward and slammed the bat into Robert's stomach.

"You call that a swing?" Robert said, suppressing the nausea that welled from his stomach. "Bet you never played ball, did you? You swing a bat like a palsied gomer!"

"Let's see how the all-star likes strike two!" Fox swung a harder blow into Robert's abdomen.

"And three … and four … and five …" Fox yelled, and commenced grunting and battering Robert's belly repeatedly.

Glad to be distracting the not-so-strong Fox from beating Guillermo, Robert tightened his stomach against each blow, his mind going back to when he was seven. His stepfather would come home drunk and angry, and Robert would immediately start messing with him to keep him from his mother and little brother. His goal was to tire the ogre out before he began whaling on them. He grew adept at dodging, but knew enough to let himself get caught before the man gave up. The blows he took then to his stomach convinced him to strengthen those muscles. He learned about sit-ups and core work even at that tender age, and he did those exercises until he couldn't do another one. Soon he noticed his stepfather's stomach blows didn't hurt as much.

When Robert wouldn't cry, his stepfather pounded him some more, becoming too exhausted to beat anyone else.

Fox was sweating and swearing now as he swung time and time again into Robert's abdomen. Robert could feel his six-pack muscles there getting sorer and sorer, and the rapidity of the blows made it almost impossible for him to try any leg-lock maneuver. He needed a break, a slip in Fox's concentration. Fox was no fool, though. He knew Robert's dangling legs could be weapons, and he was careful to stay out of their range as he batted away.

But nobody could break him. He'd die of internal bleeding before he ever gave up.

His stepfather had conditioned him well.

Fox's arms were already getting tired. He was taking more and more time between blows.

"You're not fooling me," Fox said. "I know you're hurting. I can keep this up until your liver bursts, or I can just give you a C-section." He reached down his left leg to an ankle sheath and pulled out a fierce-looking knife. He twisted the blade back and forth two inches from Robert's eyes.

Robert didn't flinch.

He felt his abs catch fire.

They were holding, though. Just as he knew they would.

Robert darted a glance at Guillermo between blows. Guillermo was listening to something.

What?

Then Robert heard it.

Distant gunfire.

Guillermo's head came up slow and strong. On full alert, ready for battle.

Fox put the knife back inside the ankle sheath and slammed Robert's gut one more time.

And Robert screamed as if he were being eviscerated, startling Fox. A big grin slowly filled Fox's face as Robert swung back from the blow toward him.

The gunfire came closer, further startling Fox.

With all the agonizing energy he could muster, Robert swung his body up and kicked Fox in the chest toward Guillermo, who knifed up and caught Fox's neck between his legs, squeezing the blood from Fox's neck and fracturing his first and second cervical vertebrae.

The bat clattered to the floor of the platform, as useless now as Fox's brain.

Guillermo vaulted off Fox's lifeless shoulders to get his legs over the holding rail above him. From that upside-down position, he unlatched the rope from the hook that held his wrists and dropped onto the platform as deftly as a cat. He pulled the knife from Fox's ankle sheath and cut the ropes that held his wrists together.

"I didn't know you still had it in you," Robert said.

With an ear-piercing screech, Guillermo pulled on Fox's legs and swung him over the platform's edge.

And watched him fall.

Amid the crack of gunfire and screams of the wounded, Robert could hear the corpse thud in the courtyard.

"Maybe if you had been a little quicker on the ball," Guillermo said, standing and dusting his hands, "and didn't play around so long with that sad excuse for a little-leaguer, we would've been out of here sooner." Guillermo reached up and cut Robert's ropes.

Robert felt instant relief. He rubbed his wrists and arms vigorously. The center of his body was screaming with every movement, but the soreness lessened slightly with each breath.

This too will pass.

The gunfire, no longer distant, had turned constant. Guillermo crept to the edge of the platform and scanned the horizon.

"What's going on?" Robert asked.

"It's Armando."

"You can tell just by the gunfire?"

"Trust me," Guillermo said. "I know how the kid fights."

"Let's get some guns and help them out."

"Stray bullets. Stray bad guys. Let's just sit it out a while. Armando's got it pretty much taken care of."

"It's not in my nature to just sit."

"Just listen for a minute."

Robert stopped at the top of the stairwell.

The battle sounds were quieting rapidly.

Then utterly.

Armando's shout drifted up. "Father! Robert!"

"Up here," Guillermo yelled, waving his arms, a huge smile splitting his face. "Armando! We're good. Well done, Son."

"It's safe to come down, sir."

By the time Robert and Guillermo made it down the limestone stairs, Armando was releasing the young villagers from their makeshift prison.

All the guards were dead.

"What about the surgeons?" Guillermo asked.

"Down below," Armando said. "We got them. We'll take them prisoners when they can walk. Couple of them got hurt pretty badly. It's what happens when you resist us."

"How are the kids?" Robert asked.

"They're good. Medics came along with us. Taking care of them."

The kids all looked scared, but were chirping to each other volubly since getting out of their cage.

"Good work, Armando," Guillermo said. "I'm proud of you, Son. But our village—how many were killed?"

"What?" Armando asked, shocked.

"Dr. Fox escaped," Robert said. "You knew that, right?"

"No! We left soon after you did. I know you said to stay, but I went ahead and recruited people to back you up."

"Fox had a GPS in his boot," Robert explained. "His buddies came and rescued him and, according to him, burned our village."

Tears burst from Armando's eyes and he doubled over, trying to catch his breath. Guillermo patted him on the shoulder.

"Let's go see, Son. Let's see how much truth there is in what that fucking weasel told us."

CHAPTER 39

The village had been torched.

The old plaza, ringed by decimated huts, was now filled with charred debris. People searched through the tangled black heaps for anything salvageable.

Robert, still sore from the beating he had endured and the trek to the village, felt dread at the thought of finding Mel's mutilated corpse.

What will I tell his wife when she finally comes out of her coma?

In the far corner of the village stood a makeshift hospital with a few people taking care of the casualties.

Robert broke into a slow, painful trot. Soon the rotund figure of one of the caregivers struck him as familiar. He started running full tilt.

Mel!

Robert's former boss was taking care of a number of children, salving their burns and bandaging their wounds. Robert called out his name, and Mel, looking up, waved wildly. He ran a few steps to meet Robert in a bear hug that nearly knocked both of them over.

"Aw man," Mel said. "I'm so glad to see you!"

"I thought you were dead. Fox said he'd killed you."

"Fox? The man's a walking lie. He should have his mouth sewn shut."

"Nothing he can do now," Robert said.

"Jesus, you killed him?"

"He was working me over with a bat. Guillermo got him in a chokehold. His cousin hyenas have him."

Guillermo limped up to them, followed by a few of the kids from Kundal. "Okay, enough talking. Some of the prisoners need medical attention."

"Absolutely." Mel took one of the boys by the hand and led him toward the infirmary.

Guillermo walked behind Mel. Upon entering the hut, he stopped and kneeled down where a little girl lay whimpering, her burned leg exposed.

"Here's some ointment." Mel tossed a pack to Guillermo, who immediately began cooing to the girl and dabbing on the salve.

Robert joined them in tending the wounded and got the story from Mel as they worked: a few hours after Armando and his crew left the village, Fox's cronies came and killed the kid guarding him.

"That motherfucker," Robert interjected with a sharp pang.

"I know," Mel said. "I was in the woods practicing my archery at the time, and that poor kid was the first corpse I saw coming back. From what I could piece together, the marauders pulled Fox with them into the woods, leaving two guards behind who just started a shooting spree. Annihilated the whole village. One with a machine gun, the other with a goddamn flamethrower. Some of us were able to escape, but some ..." He pointed to a mound of earth over a mass grave.

"What about those folks?" Robert glanced over at the long line of villagers still waiting for medical attention.

"We've already triaged them," Mel explained. "Mostly just cuts and bruises from running in the jungle."

Robert took a deep breath and looked around.

The village was destroyed.

This was my fault.

His chest threatened to explode.

"We should've killed him," Robert muttered between clenched teeth. "We should've chopped his fucking feet off and fed them to the fire. It's *my* fault."

Mel wiped his face, smearing charcoal sweat across his cheeks. "That's not true," he said. "Don't go there. No time for that." He helped a newly bandaged boy up from the cot. He gave him a gentle whack on the butt and the boy laughed and ran off.

Guillermo, with his usual perfect timing, handed Robert a towel. Robert wiped his teary eyes. Guillermo watched him, and then said gently, "We both fucked up."

"No." Robert began pacing. "You had a gut feeling that Fox was bad news. I never should have gone against your orders. We never go against our gut—you taught me that!"

"They would still have found him with the GPS, still razed the village. That's where we fucked up. You and me both. Shouldn't have been fighting over whether to kill him or not."

"We should've stripped him and burned his clothes before he entered our village."

"It's nobody's fault." Mel waved to the next villager in line. "Come in, amigo. Let me help you out."

Robert and Guillermo stared grimly at each other in silence.

Guillermo's eyes darkened. "Nobody comes to our house and gets away with this."

Robert stood still, thinking.

Joaquin was on his way to Guatemala City. All they had to do was find him.

But killing him wasn't going to be enough. He wanted to do something bigger.

Mel, sensing something in the air between them, drifted over.

"We find Joaquin," Robert said. "All his connections."

"The whole web of corruption," Guillermo said. "Everyone involved in the organ trade."

"Tear it down."

"Burn it all."

"Are you guys crazy?" Mel said. "These guys are armed. They're incorporated. They're in bed with the military, with the politicians, with the biggest blood-sucking corporations in the world. Take them out? You two? You have to get the authorities in on this."

"Listen to yourself," Robert said. "The authorities? You mean the military, the politicians, the industry giants?"

"The police," Mel shot back. "Hell, I don't know—the American embassy, the CIA."

"The authorities right now are the major part of the problem," Guillermo said.

"Part of the triad of corruption," Robert said.

"That's right," Guillermo said. "We need to firebomb the triad. The military, the corrupt judges, the organ dealers. The network funding all this illicit shit and ruining our country."

"But that's the network of criminals we can't take down," Mel said. "They're too powerful! The network is a fact of life. It's like death and taxes. It can't be weeded from the earth. People have tried throughout history. Even the Freemasons, with their hocus-pocus secret-society connections, have failed. It's the military-industrial complex. It's prostitution.

War. Drugs. Weapons. Bodies for money. It's the way of this world."

"It's the way of the world to fight for justice, Mel," Robert said.

"You two against the Mongolian hordes?"

"We're two people with nothing to lose." Guillermo looked right at Robert.

Robert nodded back.

This was not about Sharon.

Not that he could forget her. Not that she wouldn't linger in every sweet-smelling breath he took, in every free and clear thought that graced his brain. If he made it out of this one, he'd go straight to her, right back to New York City.

If not, then …

So be it.

He'd have nightmares the rest of his life if he left Guillermo now. With or without Robert, Guillermo was going after Joaquin and his network.

The very certainty of this immediately put Robert's warrior mind into action. Finding the people affiliated with Joaquin was doable. Guatemala City was small and navigable.

Confidence subdued Robert's rage and helplessness. A balanced clarity began clicking away in his mind. He could almost imagine Sharon whispering behind it all.

Finish what you started and come back to me.

"What about you, Mel?" Robert asked. "You're helping so much here, but I know you want to get back to your wife."

"I can't abandon these people."

"Guillermo and I are leaving—" Robert turned to his mentor. "When?"

"Tomorrow morning," Guillermo said. "We'll pack up those who need further medical care and take them with us to Guatemala City. Armando will escort you back with Ernesto."

"I'm going with you, Father." Armando stepped closer, his fists bunched up. "This time, I'm not giving you a choice."

Guillermo opened his mouth to object but shut it again.

"Like father, like son," Robert said.

"Okay." Guillermo placed his palm on Armando's light-bearded cheek. "You're ready."

"Thank you," Armando said.

Guillermo looked into his son's eyes, nodded, and took his hand away.

Robert stared at the horizon, toward Guatemala City. He found himself smiling.

Revenge will be sweet.

PART 3

Drug Trafficking Statistics:

- *Drug trafficking in Guatemala and Mexico generates tens of billions of dollars annually.*[12]

- *Guatemala's strategic location makes it a critical drug transit hub. Situated between Colombia and the U.S., Guatemala lies at one of the busiest drug-trafficking corridors in the world.*[13]

- *Illicit economies in Guatemala are estimated to equal up to one-fifth of GDP when including drugs, contraband, and corruption proceeds.*[14]

- *Since 2006, more than 50% of homicides in Guatemala have been linked to organized crime and drug trafficking, particularly in border and coastal regions.*[15]

- *Cartel violence in Guatemala has included large-scale massacres. In May 2011, approximately 200 armed members of a drug cartel stormed a cattle ranch in northern Guatemala, tied up 27 farmworkers—including women—and brutally executed them. This massacre was one of the bloodiest episodes in Guatemala's recent history of cartel violence.*[16]

---

[12] *U.S. Drug Enforcement Administration — National Drug Threat Assessment Reports*

[13] *United Nations Office on Drugs and Crime (UNODC) — Global Study on Homicide*

[14] *International Crisis Group — "Guatemala: Drug Trafficking and Political Power"*

[15] *Human Rights Watch. World Report 2023: Guatemala. New York: HRW, 2023.*

[16] *BBC News. "Guatemala Massacre: 27 Killed on Farm in Peten Province." 15 May 2011.*

CHAPTER 40

Robert took a slow sip of his flat beer and grimaced. It had a faint petroleum aftertaste.

Another seedy bar in downtown Guatemala City.

From his cracked vinyl barstool, he stared into the mirror before him. It was grimy and blotched but gave him a good view of the murky room. The air smelled like an old boot someone had used as an ashtray.

Their mustachioed cab driver had told them this dive was *the* place for "fun girls who were really girls." Wink, wink.

In other words, sex-trade children.

"Highly recommended," the cabbie had added. "Oil people, bankers, nice suits, Americanos, Arabs with head wraps, mucho money. No police. I drive you there? For tiny fee?"

Robert told the driver to drop them off at a hotel near there. Mel went about getting a ticket for the red-eye to New York. Guillermo, expecting a showdown in the near future, withdrew to his room to get some rest. Armando went out to nose around for word on the street about Joaquin. Robert quickly showered and shaved, put on clean casuals, and went to the bar to see if the prostitutes there might lead him up the chain of command to Joaquin.

Robert gritted his teeth and took a big gulp of the rank beer, hoping it would snap the Sharon loop running through his head. Every other minute, it seemed, his mind drifted to the safe deposit box in the city's bank that held his cellphone and computer.

To call or e-mail her.

The fantasies varied but Sharon was the constant, and contact with her was their driving force. He wanted to hear her voice. He wanted to tell her how much he missed her. He wanted her to surprise him, to move him, to tell him she missed him.

That wasn't an option. He needed to concentrate. This mission had more dangers than all the gang territories in New York. There wasn't a corner, alley, or dive in Guatemala City that didn't have eyes, ears, fists, and weapons servile to Joaquin. Despite his display of bravado for Mel, Robert knew the odds for success against the monstrously tentacled network were negligible.

Go to the bank, Robert.

Say good-bye to her.

Robert took another gulp and shuddered. He got the bartender's grudging attention, ordered a shot of mezcal and reconned the mirror again.

He counted five overly flirtatious women in too-short, too-tight outfits scattered throughout the room.

Pros. Too old.

Where are the young ones? This is supposed to be a place where you can get the youngest girls. That's my best shot at getting the intel I need.

The bartender slammed down a shot glass of mezcal before him. Robert downed it, took a quick gulp of beer, and eyed the room again via the mirror.

Start with drugs and fan out to arms dealing and slavery. And all roads now lead to organ trafficking.

To Joaquin.

Robert spotted the girl as she came through a beaded doorway.

She was maybe thirteen, dressed in a tight black skirt and tan heels that she obviously wasn't used to wearing. She took three wobbly steps, then put a hand against a table to keep from falling. The man at the table had a slow-squirming older vixen on his lap. He looked up at the much younger girl with happy expectation. Still recovering from her near fall, the girl turned up the corners of her mouth and showed her teeth in a way that reminded Robert of a nerdy kid who'd been told to smile for a school picture. The woman on the man's lap made a snake-ugly face at the girl and hissed "*Vete!*"

The girl teetered away on her spiked heels, looking as if she might burst into tears. Flustered, she leaned against the nearest wall. After taking some deep breaths and reaching down to rub her ankles, she adjusted her posture, parted her lips in what she probably had been told was a sexy expression, and glanced around with a phony smoldering gaze.

It didn't take long for a man to approach her. Robert could hear an American accent through the man's halting ridiculous Spanish.

A businessman, probably advertising.

He looked to be in his mid-fifties and wore brand new jeans and a pressed shirt.

Promising.

Robert signaled the bartender. "*Un mezcal mas.*"

The businessman grabbed the girl's elbow and pushed his beer belly into her hip. Robert saw her inch away, then instantly readjust and make a strained effort to pretend she liked the oaf.

As Robert took his time finishing his beer and shot, he noted they were conversing in short phrases, accompanied by raised eyebrows and awkward laughs of incomprehension. After five minutes riffing this pallid jazz, the couple stopped making noises at each other and left the bar.

Showtime.

Robert paid for his drinks, left the bartender an insulting tip, and sauntered after them.

The girl's shoes and tight skirt slowed their progress, and the American clutched her in a creepy avuncular way, letting his hands slide to her adolescent butt from time to time, squeezing and rubbing its scant curve vigorously.

Robert shadowed them easily through the graffiti-splattered downtown streets. The whole scene infuriated him—not only the shameless animalism of the man, but also the decrepitude of the city. Even a few years ago, when he'd last been in Guatemala City, it had been a thrumming metropolis brimming with hope, trying to recover from the Civil War. New restaurants and businesses lined the reconstituted streets.

Now there was rampant poverty, pollution, and garbage everywhere you turned. Robert felt the mezcal turn in his stomach. He couldn't believe how quickly the place he had come to call his home away from home had spiraled into such a shithole. Sometimes it seemed as if the worst of humanity had taken over everything inspiring on earth.

Robert shrugged the thought off as he made his way into a narrow alley and came upon a nodded-out youth being licked by a friendly dog. The German shepherd looked up as Robert stooped and held the back of his hand to the dog's cold wet nose, getting a lick himself.

"Taking good care of him?" Robert whispered, and the dog seemed to nod, making Robert smile for the first time all night. Out of the corner of his eye he spied his target couple slinking into the dark entrance of a decrepit hotel.

He scratched behind the dog's ears, then lifted the boy's eyelids, one at a time, growing alarmed. He took his pulse.

Jesus Christ!

The kid was dead.

Heroin overdose. Another casualty of the drug war.

A light went on in the building the couple had just entered.

Second floor.

Giving the dog's head a final scratch, Robert clambered up the fire escape of the small abandoned building across from the hotel's entrance. Its roof was littered with hypodermics, shell casings, junk-food wrappers, used condoms crawling with insects, and a half-eaten burger writhing with maggots.

There were no blinds on the lit window, and Robert could clearly see the couple standing by the side of a ratty bed. The man started groping the girl like someone trying to fight his way out of a suffocating airbag. She fought to get free of him and finally drove a spiked heel down on his instep, which made him howl loudly enough for Robert to hear.

He came at her again, and she scrambled around the bed to keep it between them. She put out her hand to him, as if demanding money first.

Shaking his head, he crawled across the bed toward her.

Robert could faintly hear her shrieking voice. "*Dinero!* Money first!"

The man grabbed her cheap rayon blouse and ripped its front, exposing a light green bra over just-budding breasts. She shrieked again and cowered in a corner. He came at her like a drunken bear and grabbed her by the throat, immobilizing her horrified face. Robert unhooked his short bow from the lining of his long leather coat and strung it with one of the arrows hidden in the lining of the coat's other side. As he was gauging his shot, the room's door burst open and a muscled man in a white tank top entered with a gun.

The pimp.

Perfect! He'll have all the information I need.

The American tore his hand from the girl's throat and raised both hands, clearly whining something like, "Don't shoot!"

Robert fired his first arrow. It splintered the glass and went deep into the pimp's bulging bicep.

The girl started screaming. The pimp dropped the gun and started yelling obscenities. The American stood stupefied with his hands up, his unbuckled pants crumpling to his ankles and revealing flabby thighs the color of a fish belly.

Robert had already anchored a coiled zip line to the roof's brick chimney and snapped its other end to his next arrow's triangular tip. He lifted the bow perfectly and shot the tethered arrow through the broken window into the room's doorframe.

And away we go.

As he slid down the slight angle toward the window, he felt a slight nostalgia for his Manhattan vigilante days. He twisted his body as his legs passed through the jagged glass, getting only one small rip in his coat pocket before landing in a deft tumble on the scratchy hotel rug. The girl was still screaming. The pimp struggled with the arrow in his arm, muttering under his breath.

The American pulled up his pants and yelled, "What the fuck!" His eyes grew wide as saucers while Robert slowly rose to his full intimidating stature holding the gun the pimp had dropped.

"Shut up!" Robert demanded.

"You're American, too," the man gasped. "Thank God!"

Robert took two quick steps and with his free hand double-punched the guy in the nose and jaw. The man began yowling and fell to his knees, both hands over his bloody, broken face. His nose was shattered, as were part of his maxilla, orbital floor, and mandible. Robert grabbed him by the shirt collar, swung him into the hallway, and shouted, "If I ever catch you child-molesting again, I'll shoot your balls off."

The man got himself on all fours and stared up at Robert, frozen in fear.

"Go!" Robert screamed. The man stumbled frenetically along the hall before he disappeared with fading whimpers down the stairwell.

Robert strode back into the room and stuck the end of the gun into the pimp's nose. The pimp's eyes were squeezed shut and he kept chanting, "*Hijo de puta! Me duele!*"

"Yeah, I bet it hurts." Robert pulled the gun away and turned to the girl. She was hyperventilating with a glassy look in her eyes. Robert picked up the short coat the American had left and gently covered the girl with it. He told her in Spanish that everything was going to get better for her now. She seemed to come out of a trance at his touch and looked up at him with teary eyes, like a little girl who had been lost and finally found her father. Robert's chest flooded with warmth.

He took the fat wallet from the coat, pulled a thick stack of hundred dollar bills from it, and handed all the money to her. Her tears stopped. Her panting turned to a dawning rush of new hope, then slowed to sighs of relief. He told her to get on a bus, leave the city, and start a new life somewhere with friends and family if she had them.

"Si," she kept nodding. "Gracias!"

It looked as if she knew exactly where she'd go, and it wasn't going to be a world of more abuse.

"*Andale.* Get going," he told her. She kissed his cheek and stepped over to the pimp, who looked at her with a pained frown.

She kicked him in the shin.

Hard.

He yowled and raised his unwounded arm to strike her, then stopped as Robert lifted the gun.

She wriggled her fingers goodbye to Robert and walked tentatively toward the door. She kicked off her spike-heeled shoes and ran from the room with the grace of a colt.

"I need a doctor," the pimp screamed in Spanish. "Get this thing out of my arm!"

Robert looked out the window. There was a little crowd gathering, some with lit cellphones to their ears.

Not much time.

He picked up one of the heel spikes. "Who sold you that girl?"

"I'm not talking until I see a doctor," the pimp spluttered.

Robert put the end of the spike directly into the pimp's eye and pushed him back against the wall.

"I'm not going to ask you again," Robert said. "The next word out of your mouth will be a name or you're going to lose your vision."

Real fear had now replaced the man's macho pose. He yelled out, "Name's a secret! No one says."

"But you've heard rumors," Robert insisted, pushing the spike in more. "In a few more seconds your lens is going to implode."

"I got her from one of my cousin's friends. He works at the nightclub!"

"What nightclub?"

"Club Kali," the pimp said.

Robert stared at the man, satisfied he was telling the truth. He pulled the spike away.

"Thanks, asshole." Robert grabbed the arrow and yanked it out.

The man fainted.

Robert pulled the other arrow from the doorframe, detached the zip line, stowed both arrows back in his coat lining, and dashed from the room, down the stairs, and into the alley, where he fired the gun three times into the air. The chattering clump of people scattered. No one bothered to look at him.

Robert heard a bark, and there was the German shepherd pawing his pant leg, looking up.

"Hey, buddy." Robert was surprised by how glad he was to see the animal. "Not afraid of gunshots? Good boy."

Robert hurried up the fire escape to the roof and collected his zip line and short bow. When he returned, the dog was waiting for him, like a serious sentry.

"What do you say you and I go clubbing? And I'll call you Doc?"

A short whimper sounded like a definite yes.

Robert laughed and made his way from the alley, stepping over the dead boy. The dog gave the corpse one last sniff, then sped after Robert.

CHAPTER 41

Robert stood outside the entrance to Club Kali with his new companion by his side. He scanned the windows and rooftops, noting the distances between buildings and taking information from the ambient noise.

A fairly quiet location.

Pedestrians and streetlights sparse.

Heavy metal music screeched from behind the club's heavy iron doors.

Robert dropped to one knee and rubbed Doc's scruff. "Why don't you hang here and have a smoke while I tend to business inside? I won't be long."

Doc raised his eyebrows.

Robert grinned and stood. Doc dug at the ground.

"Stay," Robert said.

Doc immediately sat and began panting and looking around.

"Good boy." Robert walked down the five steps to the club door. A discreet engraved gold sign above the entrance read:

Club Kali
Members Only
No Solicitors

He pounded on the door as if he were expected.

A man who looked strikingly similar to The Three Stooges' Curly, except twice his size, opened the door. "I don't know tonight's fucking password," Robert said, "and neither does Joaquin, but he told me if the goon at the door gives me any trouble to use this." Robert pulled out the pimp's gun and casually scratched the doorman's cheek with it.

"I could bite your ear off before you pull the trigger," the man said in a surprisingly high voice.

Robert laughed and poked the oaf in the eyes with two fingers of his free hand.

"Christ. That fucking hurts!" The man bent over and massaged his eyes with his huge paws.

"Oh, sorry," Robert said. "I didn't know. It's funny when The Stooges do it."

"Christ, I can barely see anything!"

"Mind if I come in now?"

"Jesus fucking Christ!"

"Thank you. I'll just borrow this." Robert took the pain-racked man's headset and his cellphone. "Stay, okay?" The man nodded vigorously. "Good boy. You don't tell anyone about this, and I won't tell Joaquin. We good?"

"Just get the fuck away from me."

Robert strode down a short hallway and up a flight of stairs, the music growing louder with every step. He swept through a double door into a ballroom-size arena, and the drums and bass pounded in his head along with the brackish clamor of a mob shouting to be heard above the tunes. Waves of bobbing heads rippled the dance floor. The people all had a look of money and the disregard for normalcy that wealth enabled. A cluster of wild-eyed women swayed in hula skirts, pearls, and nothing else. Some men wore tuxedos and others wore white tank tops.

Robert in his dark coat fit right in.

He began to dance in place, a defense against the assault of the music. He moved in a tai chi way, letting the music in instead of resisting it, ducking and diffusing when the sound blast grew too great. As he let his body go, he took ear plugs from his pocket and stuck them in his ears in what he made look like a weird but graceful dance move.

He liked to dance, and Guillermo had taught him from his first martial-arts lesson that rhythmic motion is the secret to all action in the space-time continuum. For many years now Robert had worked to keep mental and physical movement synchronized with his breath and the beat of his heart. At first he had to concentrate intensely on it, but now it was his template, the basic structure that supported all he did.

And he danced superbly.

Robert felt the elation grow as he moved through the milling crowd, no one minding his solo act, as quite a few were dancing by themselves. Sometimes he'd stop to dance with another soloist or a couple or join a threesome or small circle, always moving on after a bit. His panther grace and full-bodied expressiveness garnered happy looks as he wove among and connected with the other dancers.

All the time, of course, he was getting the lay of the land.

He saw one of three bartenders talking to a young couple overtly massaging each other's butts. The bartender pointed to a tat-covered bouncer in front of a staircase at the side of the bar.

The couple sidled toward the bouncer and whispered to him. He nodded robotically and spoke a phrase that Robert lip-read as *doscientos*. The young woman wriggled her hand out of her partner's pants clutching two bills, which the guard grabbed. The woman went up first, the man close behind, his hand pressing against her ass.

Just sex rooms up there. Rich people partying.

They're getting their drugs from somewhere else around here.

But where?

Clubs were perfect for major criminals to do their business. Loud, dark, discreet. The ideal place to buy drugs, order weapons, bid on prostitutes.

Robert swayed up to the bar and stopped. "Good moves there," the bartender said, grinning.

Robert smiled back. "Point me to some Ecstasy, and I'll really show you moves."

"Hey, yank. You a rookie here? All I know is drink. Get you anything?"

"C'mon, amigo. Who do I have to blow around here to get some blow?"

"Tell you what," the bartended laughed. "Kiss my ass and I'll give you some tequila."

"Straight up," Robert said. "No worm."

"You dance like Travolta." The barman filled a gold-rimmed shot glass, "but you dress like Columbo."

"You like the American shows," Robert said.

"What's the option? Spanish soaps?"

"I suppose so." Robert hoisted the drink. "Gracias."

The bartender muttered something from the corner of his mouth as he walked off to serve other customers.

Robert tossed down the drink and was startled by his reflection in the mirror. There was a thin red-smudged line on his cheek from his zip-line entrance through the window, not to mention the torn pocket on his plaster-dusted coat. But more alarming was the killer look on his soot-speckled face.

To his right, a handsome guy with oily hair hovered over a blank-eyed twenty-something woman, calling her *Conchita* as she chugged a full bottle of beer. On his left, a very drunk gray-haired woman in a satin dress and a tiara was flanked by two men in pastel suits, each leaning in to her with a hand on her thigh.

Robert turned his attention back to the mirror, studying the scene behind him. After a half a minute his attentive eyes caught a furtive movement across the room. A tall slouching thirty-year-old with a Hitler moustache had emerged from the kitchen looking about warily as he made his way past the sex-floor bouncer to a man by the VIP elevator. The two shook hands in a prolonged way.

Palming off a packet of drugs.

Then they went into a token bro-hug, during which the elevator man slipped something into the deliveryman's coat pocket.

Cash.

The liveried man stabbed the elevator button and got in as the delivery guy headed back into the kitchen.

Follow the money.

Robert rose from his barstool and began a tricky little shuffle step toward the kitchen. With the swinging of the door, the dance floor's gaiety and wild abandon morphed into the urgent clatter of chefs, busboys, dishwashers, and waiters rushing to keep up with their orders. Right inside the door was a stack of wooden crates filled with large cans of tomato sauce. Robert picked a crate up and walked straight through the kitchen. A diminutive chef looked at him quizzically and held up his hand in a stop gesture.

"*Inventorio.*" Robert just kept walking ahead. The chef, sweating and bedraggled as he filled five plates on the table before him, shooed Robert on.

Robert didn't see the tall messenger anywhere in the kitchen. He could see only one other exit door. He used his hip to bump it open and carried the crate into a narrow, empty hallway. After a sharp turn, he found himself in an even narrower passageway, at the end of which was the deliveryman. He was smoking a cigarillo in front of a heavy, iron door.

"*Que pasa?*" Robert said, coming up to him and setting the crate down.

"The fuck you want, Americano?"

"Your voice," Robert said and grabbed the man's protruding larynx and squeezed. "A Hitler mustache? Really?" The man made a quiet noise like motor oil glugging from a can. "How many people behind this door? Show me with your fingers."

The man tried futilely to twist out of Robert's iron grip, his mouth flapping for air, but he didn't lift his hand. Robert's free hand picked up the guy's right hand and bent it back, threatening to fracture his radius and ulna.

The man let out a muffled scream.

"Answer pronto or I'll break your hand off," Robert hissed.

The Nazi look-alike nodded and lifted his other hand and spread his fingers, tucking in his thumb.

"Four?"

He nodded.

"Password? Secret knock?"

Another nod and his hand lightly slapped the wall: *tap, tap-tap, tap*.

Robert slammed the side of his fist into the man's temple—hard enough to knock him unconscious, but nowhere near the temporal artery or venous plexus to give him an intracranial bleed.

The door had a small, sliding peephole. Robert heaved the unconscious body to a standing position and tap, tap-tap, tapped on the door. When the peephole slid open, Robert quickly turned the lifeless face away, as if it were looking behind down the passageway. The peephole slid shut, and Robert dropped the body unceremoniously on the floor. He heard three bolts unlock, and as soon as the door cracked open he power-barged through like a pro linebacker jacked up on meth. The doorman stumbled backward, holding his gun hand to his smashed nose.

Robert was dancing again, this time to the fastest tempo of the night. In a graceful sweep he snatched the doorman's gun and put a bullet through his right eye. Simultaneously, he drew his pimp gun and shot the right hands and knees of the two guards standing by the desk across the room. One of them passed out immediately from the shock, the other fell to his side, mewling quietly with a hurt child's look in his eyes. Then Robert aimed both guns at the man behind the desk.

"I'll make this quick," Robert said. "I want you to tell me where I can find Joaquin."

The man remained stock-still. He stared at Robert like a snake about to strike. Then a slight ripple in the man's lower abs told Robert he was shifting his leg further under the desk.

"Stop that foot." Robert moved forward and aimed a gun at the man's knees. "Unless you want a shattered patella like your useless bodyguards."

The man froze, but his eyes veered up and to the right.

Camera!

Any minute there would be more guards. Robert needed the information.

Now.

He darted a look at the guards, now recognizing them. He had seen their mug shots on the news after a bunch of workers at a cattle ranch had been massacred by their drug cartel.

He shot the unconscious man on the floor in the jugular, then right below the aortic arch in the heart. Then he put a bullet through the lungs of the whimpering guard, causing a hemothorax, and another one through his larynx.

He turned his guns back to the man, whose amazed eyes and compulsive gulping showed that he knew Robert meant business.

"Stop stalling," Robert shouted and shot a bullet from each gun into the chair right between the man's legs.

"Don't shoot me! I'll talk!"

Robert shot again, this time nicking the fabric covering the man's crotch. The man jumped up with his hands clamped ridiculously over a spreading urine stain.

"He's in *Las Nubes.* It's all there, at the warehouse. Drugs, arms, prostitutes, organs—everything goes through there."

Robert now heard a pounding of approaching footsteps. He quickly shot the man in the kneecaps and feet.

"*Hijo de puta!*" the man screamed in agony.

"Such filthy language, Señor. You kiss your *madre* with that mouth?" Robert unzipped a pocket at the hem of his coat. He pulled out a blue titanium canister, set its timer for one minute and placed it on the ground.

"*Vete a la mierda,*" the man moaned, his swearing rapidly losing its vehemence.

"I shot you to lessen your time in purgatory." Robert aimed his zip line at the ground floor doorframe in the building across the street. His new best friend was there, looking up. He zip-lined the arrow straight and true into the cement frame.

"Me cago en la leche!" the man whined.

"You had some bad luck all right," Robert said, "and so has everyone who ever met you until me. *Adios, pendejo!*"

A gaggle of thugs stormed into the room, and Robert slid out the window. A split second after he landed, he activated his bow's powerful retracting mechanism and the zip line twanged from the window and neatly coiled back into the bow's inner packing. Robert began sprinting, and Doc was right on his heels. As they reached the main street, a reverberating explosion rattled the lampposts.

The lights dimmed.

"Mission accomplished, Doc. First leg of it anyway."

Doc started trotting toward Robert's hotel.

"Good dog!" Robert ran after him. "Let's go get ready for the real showdown."

CHAPTER 42

A whole host of weapons lay piled on the hotel bed, and Doc was sniffing each one.

"Where is Mel?" Robert asked.

"Napping," Guillermo said. "The hike took a toll on him."

Robert nodded, wondering if he should wake him up for their talk.

"This is a very special animal." Guillermo tracked Doc's delicate movements. When Robert had returned to the hotel room with Doc at his side like a brother-in-arms, Guillermo's eyes had locked onto the dog with the glow of a doting grandfather. Doc, in turn, had taken an equal shine to Guillermo, immediately going to where he sat and pressing against the man's crossed legs.

When Doc yipped, Guillermo had fed him Nutter Butter cookies purchased earlier from the vending machine down the hall. Doc wolfed them down and wagged his tail after licking the empty pack clean.

By that time, Robert had spread out his arsenal. Everything seemed okay until Robert lifted his favorite toy, his bow.

"The bow question," Guillermo said. "It's a lot to pack, Robert. Bulky. And the arrows. We have a lot of other stuff: the zip line, explosives, rocket launcher ..."

"I hate to leave it behind," Robert said.

"That's because you're in love with it," Guillermo said. "You get a pheromone rush when you rub its pearly skin."

Robert laughed. "True."

"It's urban warfare, now. No need to worry about pollution or scaring the animals."

"The animals are the traffickers, and we don't want to scare them off too soon with gun noises."

"We're using silencers." Guillermo pointed to the three Gemtech suppressors sunk in one of the pillows. Doc gave a quiet *ruff* to underscore the point.

Robert sighed.

"Leave the bow and arrows here," Guillermo said.

"Okay." Robert started filling his duffel bag with weapons, ammo, and gear. Guillermo stooped to look under the bed and pulled out another duffel. "Whoa there," Robert said. "What're you doing, old man?"

"Packing my bag."

"You're still hurt. I don't need you. It's a night op. My specialty. Right up my dark alley. You need to rest."

"There's no way I'm sitting this one out."

"You're not coming, Guillermo. I can handle this on my own."

"I don't doubt it, but I want a piece of the action."

"I'm going, too." Armando emerged from the bathroom dressed in combat black, his face tarred with glistening stripes.

Robert and Guillermo looked at each other and laughed.

"It's Shadow Man," Robert said. "He slips through the shadows like night's own ghost."

"Your face is already dark enough, Armando," Guillermo said. "No need for makeup."

"Makeup's for girls," Armando said defensively. "This is camouflage."

"War paint," Robert corrected, coming to the kid's rescue. "Gives you a good feeling, too. I know." Armando's enthusiasm gave him a lift. It reminded him of his start with Guillermo years ago. He liked the idea of a new generation of fighters. Bold, brazen, fearless.

He turned back and saw Guillermo smiling at him.

He loves Armando like this even more than I do.

With a bark, Doc jumped off the bed and headed into the bathroom for a toilet drink. The three men could hear him lapping as they continued to pack their sacks.

Armando squinted into a riflescope while Robert finished putting ammo in his shotgun, spread a map on the empty bed, and grabbed a marker.

"All right," Robert said as they flanked him, "The warehouse is here." He circled it and began making a game plan with X's, O's, and arrows. Armando and Guillermo listened with grave attention. From time to time, Guillermo added comments, peering at his son to make sure he understood.

Armando did.

Doc's whimpers interrupted them. "He's probably wondering what his assignment is," Guillermo said.

"His assignment is to stay in this room," Robert said. "We can't have him barking, giving us away."

"He won't bark," Guillermo said.

A beat passed as Robert looked at Guillermo. Robert saw the same sure truth in those eyes that warmed him when they first met.

"He does follow commands—and he's definitely not afraid of gunshots," Robert said. "Okay, we'll take him with us."

"We could always use him as a distraction." Guillermo stared down at Doc, who stared right back up, his body vibrating slightly.

"We'll have to recon how many men they have." Robert turned his attention back to the map. "I expect a lot. We might have to go in shooting."

"So every shot has to count," Guillermo said pointedly to Armando.

"You know my shooting, Father," Armando said. "Heads will explode. Hearts will get ripped. Every shot will be lethal."

"I don't want you leaving me alone on this planet." Guillermo put a hand on Armando's shoulder.

"Wherever you end up, Father, I'll end up beside you."

Guillermo nodded. "I like the readiness in your voice. And just enough fear to convince me you're assessing things realistically. Good."

"I'm not afraid to die any more than you are, Father. Mainly I want them to pay for what they did to our family and village."

"Your mom would kill me if she knew I was letting you come along on a mission," Guillermo said. "But she would understand. She always does."

Robert thought about his first meeting with Rivera, the triage nurse at the St. Jude's emergency department. Guillermo had put him in touch with her after Robert had left his elective medical rotation in Guatemala. Neither Guillermo nor Rivera talked openly about their relationship, but Robert had pieced together most of the story.

It was about sacrifice.

Rivera knew Armando would grow up to be a better person if he were raised surrounded by nature rather than by the loud noises of a tiny cramped studio apartment in Spanish Harlem.

Plus, Guillermo didn't have to go to work four times a week. He could spend every waking minute with their son.

Robert turned to Guillermo, who looked like he was holding back tears. Robert had rarely seen him so emotional. Guillermo started to speak but choked a bit on his words. He cleared his throat and said softly, "Just keep your earpiece on, Armando. We'll keep communicating. You'll know if we run into trouble."

"Got your back," he replied, with a wry smile.

Robert stared back.

My life will be in his hands.

Do I trust him?

Beads of sweat lined the young man's temples, but his breathing was steady and strong.

Robert eyed Armando head to toe.

I do.

Doc barked, shook his whole body as if he were coming out of water and pointed at the door with a barely audible growl.

"Okay, let's make these guys pay," Guillermo said.

Robert nodded. "We leave in fifteen minutes. I need to take care of something first."

CHAPTER 43

Robert found Mel on the edge of his bed, hands cradling his head.

"Hey, Mel. You okay?"

"Not really." He straightened up, wiping his face. "I keep flashing back on what happened to the village. There's like this hologram documentary of it in my head I can't shake. Damn, those guys were worse than animals. You and Guillermo were absolutely right about wanting to exterminate them, and I was an idiot for thinking otherwise."

"You're in shock, Mel, but you'll be functioning fine before long."

"I don't know, Robert."

"Listen, I can tell you from experience. The nightmare of it will melt down to hard truths soon enough. It won't ever leave you completely, though. It's knowledge we have to remember. To help us do our part. Whenever we can."

Mel squeezed his belly fat on both sides. "Wish I were in better shape—and that I had more balls. I'd go out with you all and do my part to help punish those bastards."

"I appreciate that, boss, but it's not called for at this time," Robert said. "We have enough manpower, especially now with Armando joining us."

Mel gave a nervous laugh.

"Anyway," Robert said, "you need to go back to New York and be there when your wife comes to."

"I'm going to show her I'm a changed man," Mel said. "I'll do anything to make her feel better, and nothing to cause her any more pain."

"I know."

Mel sighed. "And I can do it, too. Show her the real Mel Weiss, the one you brought out of hiding."

Robert couldn't keep from smiling, but only briefly as they both felt the seriousness of this encounter. This could be the last time they saw each other. "Have you contacted St. Jude's?" Robert asked. "To see how Francine is doing?"

"Haven't had the time," Mel said. "Soon as I get my sorry ass in motion again, I'll pack and find someplace where my phone works. I'll give Rivera a call. I'm sure she'll know the latest."

"She always does." A vision of Rivera rose in Robert's mind: standing strong and tall, listening to Sharon intensely venting concerns about a patient.

"I can't thank you enough, Robert."

"No problem, amigo."

Despite his aversion to being touched, Robert accepted Mel's hug with a solid pat on the back.

"Please be careful," Mel said. "I don't want you getting hurt."

They separated and Robert smiled again. "Don't worry, boss. We'll just keep our hearts pure, right?"

"Amen to that," Mel roared. They both laughed, then Mel grew somber. "And I mean it about letting me know if there's anything I can ever do for you. Just say the word."

"As a matter of fact"—Robert pulled a sealed envelope from his pocket—"I want you to give this to Sharon if I don't make it back to New York."

"Sure." Mel took the envelope like it might contain anthrax. "But you know you'll make it through this, right? You and Guillermo have been through worse. It's a sure thing, right?"

"Nothing's a sure thing."

"True." Mel looked nervous again.

Robert glanced at his watch and headed for the door. "I have to go. If you don't see me in New York by the weekend, give it to her, okay?"

"And say what?"

Robert found himself unable to talk. A lump bottlenecked his throat and a wave crested up from his heart into his eyes. He squeezed them shut, and the wave crashed behind his lids. He took a deep breath and exhaled, the effort sounding like water receding from the shore. He opened his eyes and wiped them quickly and found his voice half an octave lower than his usual range. "Tell her …"

"You know what, don't say anything. Just make it home. Tell her everything then."

Robert nodded, relieved. He imagined sneaking inside Sharon's apartment and surprising her. His heart ached just thinking about it.

Mel shook the envelope. "What's in here, anyway? What's the secret prize?"

"The key to my security box in New York. I gave my accountant instructions to give Sharon access to all I own. It's got the bulk of my inheritance from my grandfather. I know Sharon will find a way to get the money to those who need it the most."

"Done." Mel tossed the envelope into the open suitcase on his bed. "Now, go on. Go get those dirt bags. And make it back alive, okay?"

"Will do. Take care, friend."

"You, too. Take great care."

Robert opened the door, paused, took his room key from his pocket, and handed it to Mel. "I'm leaving my bow in my room. I want you to have it."

"No way! I know what it means to you."

"I can get another set. I want you to have it. For what this visit has been for us."

"How will I pack it? Or get it past customs?"

"The bow can be disassembled. It has its own carry bag."

"You won't need it?"

"We got firepower, grenades, and a dog." Robert walked to the doorway. "See you later, Mel."

And he shut the door behind him.

CHAPTER 44

They stood on a rooftop in a remote suburb of Guatemala.

"I count three guards on the roof." Robert stared through his high-def night-vision glasses. It was ten p.m., and the large warehouse across the street had shades across every window. Little light leaked. The surrounding buildings looked abandoned, but Robert was sure Joaquin owned the entire block.

Guillermo studied the wallet-size screen of the thermal scope aimed at the warehouse. "I count twenty-two on the first floor," he said. "These guys are like a small military, and I think we're getting their honor guard."

"Better get right to shooting then." Armando's left foot jigged up and down.

"Easy, Rambo," Robert said.

"Remember son, study your enemy with as much zeal as you would study your lover's body." Guillermo moved the scope up to read the second floor. "The more you learn, the greater your advantage."

"Yes, Father." Armando reached inside the bag and pulled out the three Gemtech suppressors. "I'll start putting the silencers on."

"Good idea," Robert said.

"Six guards on the second floor," Guillermo said, "and a tight pack of what looks like twelve prisoners. From their height I'd guess all girls, but can't say for sure."

"More fodder for their sex and organ trade," Robert said.

"And four more guards on the third floor, under the roof. Passing around a joint."

"Rifles ready," Armando said, all business now.

"Let's have them," Robert ordered, and Armando smacked a rifle into Robert's hands as precisely as a scrub nurse would pass a scalpel to a surgeon. Then another into his father's hands.

"Well done," Guillermo said. "Let's take a look then."

They all knelt, lined their suppressor-heavy barrels up on the low roof wall, and peered through the powerful scopes. "Why are they moving around so much?" Armando asked.

"I don't know," Robert snapped. Skittish movement would make the kill shots less accurate.

"They're on meth," Guillermo said. "If you look closer you can see their jaws constantly moving, grinding their teeth or jabbering."

"Damn," Robert said. "We should wait until they get more riled up."

"Agreed," Guillermo said.

"Fucking druggies," Armando said.

"It's quieter than I thought it would be," Guillermo said softly. "I'm afraid even with the suppressors, the shots might cause unwanted attention."

"Why don't we send the dog down there?" Armando suggested. "He can cause a distraction."

Guillermo nodded. "Brilliant idea."

"Yeah, perfect." Robert reached down, patted Doc on the side, and pointed to the door.

Doc sprang up from where he was curled at Robert's feet and disappeared down the stairs.

A minute later they heard loud howls erupting from the street. The main door to the warehouse slammed open and a hulk of a man in black fatigues stepped out and clapped his hands. Doc immediately stopped howling, and the man whistled to the dog.

"You take the guy on your left, Armando, I got the middle man …"

"… and I'll take the one on the right," Robert said.

All three of the roof guards were now perfect targets as they peered over their roof ledge at the dog action below. The whistling guard started clapping his hands again, chanting, "*Buen perro!*"

"Good dog, indeed," Robert whispered. "Ready. Aim."

Doc began another long howl. The guard roared with laughter, and the three roof druggies smiled and jabbed each other.

"Fire!"

As one, three loud *phhts* coughed from their rifles and the three roof guards were blown backward, dead from hollow-pointed bullets to their foreheads.

"*Dame la pata,*" the ground guard called to Doc, totally unaware of the deadly shots that had flown above him. Immediately Doc stopped yowling and trotted to the guard, his tail wagging, and lifted his paw. With a loud laugh, the guard shook it. Then Doc withdrew it and scampered through the open doorway. "Hey, come back," the man yelled jovially, chasing after, slamming the door behind him.

"What's Doc doing in there?" Robert asked, feeling more worried than he had all night.

"Infiltrating," Guillermo said without a trace of sentiment. "Like we should be doing." He shot the zip line at a slight downward angle into the roof wall across the street.

"Yeah, let's go." Robert turned to Armando. "Okay, kid. We'll hit that roof and work our way down. When we give the word," he stooped and patted the rocket launcher, "you make a hole in the building. Shake them up like an earthquake jolting a bridge at rush hour. Then get the truck and be ready to move."

"Remember to focus," Guillermo added. "Breathe deeply and get your mind in a state of flow."

"And remember our primary objective," Robert said.

"Killing Joaquin," Armando answered between gritted teeth.

"No," Robert said, shaking his head. "Getting the girls out safely."

And killing Joaquin.

With that, Robert slid across, Guillermo trailing.

CHAPTER 45

Their flashlights revealed a lot of gore on the warehouse roof: three fragmented corpses, blood and organs splayed on the light-gray cement floor. With dispatch, Robert and Guillermo stripped the bodies of ammunition and headed for the stairs. Meanwhile, Armando reeled the zip line in from across the building.

In silence they crept down the dark, narrow stairwell. Robert led, holding the Sig Sauer at his side. They paused on the landing and turned on their Bluetooth audio-enhancing earpieces. Into their ears came the blather of stoned bad guys talking about stuff they'd like to do with prostitutes.

Armando's whispery voice broke through their earbuds, overriding the stoner blather. "I read you on the landing. Infrared says two guards on your right as you enter, two on your left. All sitting. Have fun." The stupid, droning conversation of the guards came back on as Robert signaled to Guillermo: *I'll take the two on the right.*

Guillermo nodded.

At that moment, a loud jet flew overhead, ready to land at a nearby airport. Robert and Guillermo used the noisy intrusion to burst into the third-floor front room. The guards looked up curiously, irked, as if about to complain. Robert lung-shot the goon on the couch still holding in smoke from the joint he'd just dragged. The man coughed and gurgled blood through his gaping mouth before collapsing on the floor. Robert then double-tapped—chest, then head—the guard who'd been reaching toward his blown-away companion as if the only thing that mattered was to keep the joint from dropping to the floor. His jolted fingers slipped over the burning ember as his nervous system closed down and all sense of life vanished. Guillermo dispatched the other two thugs, stopping a tug-o-war over a tequila bottle. They ended up with their foreheads touching over the bottle opening.

"Aw. That's sweet," Robert whispered to Guillermo.

"Good to add art to one's work," Guillermo sallied back.

The noise from the overhead jet was now a distant whoosh. Robert spoke softly into his mini microphone. "Armando, you copy?"

"I see two orange blobs still standing. Nice work."

"Don't pop the champagne yet," Robert said. "Look below. Are the prisoners in the room by the fire-escape window?"

"Affirmative. And six guards in the room next to it."

"We're going down the fire escape. Get your rocket launcher fired up."

"Copy that."

Robert turned to Guillermo. "Let's get this thing done."

They hustled to the open window and climbed onto the fire escape. Mounds of pigeon droppings littered the steps and railings, and the parts that weren't covered were grainy with loose rust. Robert almost slipped on his first step down, and Guillermo swatted his head. "Stay Zen," he murmured. Robert rubbed his head and nodded, moving down with mindfulness this time, his breath and body joined in seamless grace, sure-footed, no more slipping.

When he reached the metal-railed landing outside the second-floor room, Robert heard the quiet chatter of the prisoners in the room behind the shaded window. "Just female voices," he whispered.

"Makes sense from their heights," came Armando's response.

"Guards?" Guillermo demanded.

"Negative," Armando said. "Not in that room. In the one next to it. Six of them. Standing. Better than the jokers upstairs."

"Fire the rocket launcher at the first floor," Guillermo ordered.

"Yes, Father."

A second later Robert heard a huge explosion and felt the building shudder.

During the ensuing aftershock—full of screams, shouts, and crashing debris—Robert broke through the window, followed by Guillermo. The prisoners inside were all females, young teens in various stages of fright and hysteria from the explosion.

The smell of smoke from the floor below grew stronger by the second. Robert spotted a girl who looked mature for her age trying to calm the girls who were on the verge of losing it completely. Then he saw Guillermo go right to her, and shout in Spanish, "We're here to help. We're getting all of you out of here."

Robert positioned himself by the door to the other room, preparing to decimate any guards coming though. Guillermo and the girl corralled the other prisoners and sent them climbing out the window and down the fire escape to the truck Armando had driven there. When Robert heard rapid machine-gun fire, he knew Armando was carrying out the next phase of the plan: gunning the ground floor, showing no mercy.

The door to the room slammed open. Robert rammed his rifle stock directly into the forehead of the hulking bearded guard who barged through, then shot a bullet that went in one ear and out the other. The falling carcass tripped up the guard pushing behind him, and Robert kicked the guard's head as he fell, knocking him unconscious. When two more guards crowded in behind them and raised their Uzis, Robert shot both of them between the eyes. The two remaining guards, who couldn't see or get past the pile-up at the door, turned and ran. Robert lobbed a grenade after them—it looped over their shoulders and exploded just as they reached its point of impact.

By this time all the girls were out the window. Robert could hear their hurried steps down the fire escape. Then the pounding shockwaves of Armando's machine gun stopped. The clanging on the fire escape ceased as well. Robert turned his head and waited for new sounds. He wondered if Armando and the prisoners had made it out.

Were they in danger?

"Girls are safe," Guillermo said.

Robert heard the sound of the truck driving away, and Armando's voice in their ears. "Taking the prisoners to the hotel. Take care of whatever I left you."

"Good job, Son," Guillermo said. "I'm proud of you. We're hitting the first floor now."

"A lot of smoke and fire down there, but I saw some figures still lurching around. Be careful."

"Always," Guillermo said.

Armando said something else but his voice broke up as he put distance between them.

Guillermo clapped Robert's shoulder with an iron grip. "Let's see if Joaquin survived."

CHAPTER 46

They opened the door to the stairwell leading to the ground floor. A cloud of thick smoke knocked them back a few steps.

"Not down there," Guillermo rasped.

Doubled over and coughing, Robert couldn't respond—he just pointed back at the fire escape. Guillermo nodded and they both staggered to the window and into the outside air. When they were halfway down, a bullet bounced off the iron rung beneath Robert's foot. An obese guard lying at the base of the stairwell with a jagged chair leg through his abdomen was trying to lift his arm again for another shot. With a jungle roar, Guillermo leapt off the fire escape onto the man's bulging stomach, causing an even louder grunt from the guard. Guillermo then jammed his Sig down the man's throat and fired. As Guillermo sprang to his feet, Robert landed neatly beside him.

They could now see into the first floor through the exploded windows. A number of men were spraying fire extinguishers throughout the large room. The air was steamy, but the red-hot fires were being put out.

Robert started to lunge forward but Guillermo's calm hand made him pause. "Let them put the fires out," he whispered.

Robert nodded. His throat felt like he had swallowed bees. "Water?" he croaked out.

"Here." Guillermo handed Robert a small liquor flask.

Robert was surprised but grateful. He never knew Guillermo to drink. He took a gulp of what he thought would be mezcal but had the taste of jalapeno turpentine. "Agh!" he sputtered, his eyes widening with sudden wetness that felt more like sweat than tears. "What the hell is this?"

"Your throat good now?" Guillermo took a swallow himself as smoothly as if he were drinking water.

Robert's throat, in fact, felt clear and clean as a waterslide now. He wiped the tears from his eyes. "Fantastic. What is that stuff?"

"Just herbs."

"Does the job. You ready?"

"Been waiting all day for this."

Robert grunted and they slunk toward the warehouse entrance. Its heavy door had been blown half off its hinges. They scurried through, weapons up. Only a few weak lights flickered, filtering through the clearing smoke in an eerie way. They could make out five shadowy figures, and the sound of the fire extinguishers stopped. No visible fires could be seen burning. Robert stalked toward three figures on the right, and Guillermo approached the two on the left.

The quiet sounds of hissing and settling debris were shattered by their guns.

They walked slowly among the destruction and the dead, hearts pounding with adrenaline, eyes alert for possible enemy fire. The ceiling above—the floor of the room where the girls had been held—had half-collapsed, dropping furniture and body parts onto the carnage below.

It was like walking through a nightmare.

Robert tried to count the number of dead, to determine if there were still any guards left who might be trouble—but the bodies were in so many pieces it was impossible.

They met over a pile of two torsos, various arms and legs, half a head, and a stove.

"No sign of Joaquin," Robert said. "At least nothing I can recognize."

"He's alive," Guillermo said, "and not far from us."

Robert looked at him somberly. It was chilling to be in the presence of his old teacher at times like this—Guillermo tuned in to a remote psychic space, his eyes flickering with some faraway fire—and Robert believed him. Joaquin was nearby.

And we have to put him away.

Forever.

Robert heard a single bark from a distance, and he broke into a trot. Guillermo followed behind closely. They ran through a doorway and found more destruction and carnage. In a far corner of the room they saw Joaquin, pinned under a smoldering door. Doc was a few feet away, growling.

Robert and Guillermo lifted it off, careful of the hot spots. Joaquin was unarmed and looked pathetic and helpless. "Thank you," he said weakly as they helped him to his feet.

Joaquin seemed to have trouble standing, but Robert could see no visible wounds or obvious injuries on him.

"Why don't you just kill me?" Joaquin asked.

"I have a few questions first," Guillermo said. "Then I'll end your miserable existence."

CHAPTER 47

"Just kill me," Joaquin yelled. "I have nothing worth living for. You've ruined everything I've ever worked for."

Guillermo aimed his gun at Joaquin's chest. Joaquin reflexively crossed his arms in front of him and moved away from the line of fire.

"Please don't shoot," Joaquin pleaded, like a child.

Robert lifted his Sig, fell to one knee, and began a three-hundred-sixty-degree assessment of his surroundings.

Something's raising the hair on my neck.

But he saw no threats as Guillermo kept laying into his former prodigy.

"You have no remorse for what you've done, Joaquin. There's still a black light in your eyes. You're not done harvesting children, stuffing what's healthy in the poor into what's rotten in the rich, turning our country and its people into your chop shop."

"You think stopping me will stop minds like mine from improving the human race?"

"Tell me about your whole organization, all your lackeys, all your outposts. We've stopped you. Now we have to stop the rest of the atrocities you've put in motion."

"You have no idea what you're up against," Joaquin said. "Even if you stop us in Guatemala, there's organ harvesting, sex trading, arm and drug dealing all over the world. You'll never put a dent in our network. We're global and replaceable—take one of us out, there are ten others waiting to take our place."

"No danger on the perimeter," Robert interjected. "He's stalling with bullshit, hoping someone will rescue him."

"Why did you turn, Joaquin?" Guillermo asked with real concern.

"I learned from you for a while," Joaquin replied, "then I learned from a greater beast—life itself."

"Because your father died from hyperkalemia?" Robert butted in. "Because he couldn't get a kidney transplant? That can't be the only reason."

"You don't know what it's like to be slapped around like that by death when you're a kid," Joaquin hollered. "It teaches you to hate. To fuck the world. My father was one of the good guys." He was on the verge of tears. "That changes a kid. Life is a fickle bitch, and if blood's the price she wants, better it be someone else's blood."

"I know what it's like to lose a parent that young—and so does Guillermo," Robert said. "But our response isn't vengeful slaughter."

"It isn't? Tell that to all the body parts lying around here."

"We do it to defend others," Guillermo said. "You do it to fatten your purse and puff up your chest."

"Don't tell me you're not proud of your violence. But you're also too proud to admit I do more good than you. That's right! I've saved hundreds of lives, whereas you've saved a measly few. I trade doomed lives for prosperous ones. The greedy millions I make in the process help me continue to make millions prosper. If you don't buy Machiavelli, then consider Darwin. Survival of the fittest."

Robert scoffed. "The devil quoting scripture. Not only are you sewing the Machiavelli label onto your bullshit material but you're also changing Darwin's primal theory. Did you even read the book? He mentions survival of the fittest only twice, but he mentions love about a hundred times."

"Love? As if that's what life is about." Joaquin shook his head. "Tell me this, Dr. McKenzie, was it love that watched kindly as my dad screamed his last twenty-four hours away? Was it tender loving care that pushed my mother into the streets of Guatemala City to beg for food and rent out her fucking birth canal so she could feed her three kids? Or are you talking about the great compassion other people showed us by holding their noses as they passed? As they treated us like garbage? I prefer life as my teacher, not love—and certainly not Guillermo's crap lessons!"

"There's no use talking to you, Joaquin," Guillermo said. "I guess there never has been."

"We've all had tough lives," Robert said. "You chose the wrong path."

"Sure," Joaquin snapped with another burst of nastiness. "But you didn't learn from your experiences. I did."

"I'm tired of this," Guillermo said. "Just tell us what you know about the network."

During the quiet that descended, a look of fury suffused Joaquin's face, and he started to lift his hand.

Guillermo shot his little finger off.

Joaquin's yowl trumped the volume of the shot as he fell to his knees, crying and gulping in pain. He yanked off his bandana and tightly bandaged his bleeding hand, his cries turning to whimpers.

Guillermo and Robert watched in grim silence. Then Guillermo shifted his aim. "Your ear next, if you make another false move. Start talking."

"Just kill me," Joaquin sniveled.

"Tell us what we want to know …" Guillermo dropped hard on the ground, a dart in his jugular.

Robert whirled in the direction the dart had come from, saw nothing, heard a *phht*, and felt a dart pierce the hollow of his throat. He wrenched it out, tried to speak but couldn't, tried to turn the gun back on Joaquin but found it hard to move, and saw Joaquin in front of him, a triumphant smile plastered on his evil face as he took the gun away.

CHAPTER 48

Joaquin grimaced with pain as he held his bloodied hand. "Did you like my sob story, Dr. McKenzie?"

Robert tried to speak but nothing came out.

"It touched your heart, didn't it? Enough for Pablo, my all-star sniper, to get the dart laced with etomidate on you."

With effort Robert ratcheted his neck to look around the room. He saw straw-sized holes in a triangle pattern at regular intervals on the walls. Each set of three had two holes on top for the eyes and one below for the blowgun.

"Pablo!" Joaquin called. "Maintain your watch while I take care of my hand." Joaquin walked over to Guillermo's supine body and kicked him in the kidney. "You're going to pay for what you've done!"

Guillermo didn't move.

"If either of them starts moving again," Joaquin instructed Pablo, "give them more toad juice."

Robert heard a slight movement behind the wall ahead of him to the left.

Eyeing Robert warily, Joaquin opened a cabinet, took out bandages and disinfectants, and expertly doctored his hand, wincing at the flashes of pain but gloating all the while at Robert.

"The truth is," Joaquin said laughing, "my mother was kind of a hag. She couldn't sell herself to a blind Viagra addict. She let my brothers and me starve. We'd go begging for food, then come home and see her staring into space. And when we cried? She'd grab a plastic bag and wrap it around our face. One time I passed out. When I woke up she was smoking a cigarette, smacking my face with a fly swatter. Ah, memories."

His hand bound with clean white bandages, Joaquin opened a drawer and pulled out two sets of handcuffs. "I expect some sparks might be sputtering back into your freeze-framed axons any second now, so let's cuff you up."

He jerked Robert's hands behind him and cuffed them, humming an aria from *Carmen*. Then he knelt by Guillermo's prone body, cuffed him the same way, tugged his head up by the hair, slammed it against the concrete floor, then lifted an eyelid and peered in.

"I'm going to enjoy torturing you." Joaquin slammed Guillermo's head once more on the floor. He stood and sauntered toward Robert.

"Sadist," Robert managed to say.

Joaquin laughed.

Robert felt a tingling begin in his limbs, like icepick pricks. He tried curling his toes and found he could. He felt a squeamish movement in his stomach and a gag reflex in his throat as he noted Guillermo's new head wound slowly pooling red onto the white-painted concrete.

"Fuck it," Joaquin said, picking up Robert's Sig. "He's no fun any more." He put the barrel to the side of Guillermo's head. "*Adios, anciano*!"

"Wait!"

Joaquin turned to Robert with a delighted smile. "Can't handle seeing your teacher die like a pig?"

Robert slowly stomped his right foot, feeling pins and needles rocket through it. He felt his throat and tongue loosen, but he didn't want to let Joaquin know how much better he was beginning to feel. "Let's … f-f-fight … you … f-f-fucking … p-p-pussy."

"Fight you? Hardly!" Joaquin laughed aloud, but then his face flushed. "A little payback for what you guys did today? A little recreation? Yeah. So first a little recreational drug." He slipped a small glass bottle from his pocket, straightened its built-in straw, and snorted. "Fuck yeah!" he howled, tilting his head back and wiping his nose rapidly.

Robert had more time to thaw.

"Okay," Joaquin said, "let's do this."

Robert focused his gaze on Joaquin, feeling his reviving heart start to pump the natural high of pure adrenaline into his bloodstream.

"Uncuff me," Robert said, staring at his wrist.

"I have the handicap of a maimed hand." Joaquin picked up a long surgeon's scalpel. "So I need to compensate for it."

"I'm barely mobile!"

"It's a party"—Joaquin grinned, swishing the scalpel before him—"not a contest."

CHAPTER 49

Robert struggled upright. His gaze avoided the waving scalpel and focused instead on the man's navel as Joaquin inched forward.

Arms and heads can feint, but the belly never lies.

And sure enough, Joaquin looked left and plunged the blade right.

Robert tracked the movement with the accuracy of a sniper and stepped aside in time, despite his still-sluggish legs. He immediately began bouncing on his toes to further activate his kinetic energy. It took Joaquin a half-second to recover from the overreach of his lunge, and Robert took advantage of this imbalance by hip-bumping him three staggering steps aside. Without pause, he followed his faltering opponent as nimbly as he could and kicked at his bandaged hand, connecting solidly. Joaquin yelled in outrage, as if shocked by his opponent's bad sportsmanship, and Robert took another half step and slammed the hand again.

More yelling.

He moved in for a third kick, saw Joaquin's eyes look at the sidewall and his head nod.

Robert dropped to his knees quickly enough for the dart to sail through the hair on the top of his head. It clanged off the metal medical cabinet.

Robert noted where the dart man stood, then focused on his opponent. Joaquin shook his wounded hand for a moment before advancing remorselessly, holding the scalpel in front of him with his good hand.

"Duck!" came Guillermo's voice.

Robert did. Another dart sailed past, barely missing Joaquin.

"Goddamn it, Pablo! Watch where you're blowing that thing," Joaquin barked, still coming closer. "Dart the old man!"

From the corner of his eye, Robert saw Guillermo start rolling himself against the wall, leg-hooking a capsized chair in front of him for protection.

Joaquin began to walk around Robert like a shark circling his prey. He took a step forward and slashed. Robert again dropped to the ground, this time sweeping his right leg forward to trip his opponent. As he fell, Joaquin cut Robert deep above the right knee.

Robert didn't have time to stanch the wound. He lurched up, feeling a sickening weakness in his leg that burned and made him stumble. Joaquin bellowed like a gored bull as he got himself upright and gave Robert's bleeding knee a painful blow.

"Don't shoot, Pablo!" he yelled, his coked-up eyes jittering angrily at Robert, who was bent over gasping from the kick and trying to put his cuffed hand over the deep cut. "This *puta* is mine now." Joaquin rocked back, then stepped forward with another kick at the wound, while his scalpel hand roundhoused toward Robert's ear. Robert spun in the direction of the roundhouse, outrunning both the kick and the jab. Joaquin twirled one-hundred-eighty-degrees, connecting only with empty air. Robert slammed himself into the wall, right at a pyramid of holes. He heard a faint squeal and saw two dark eyes recede from the top two.

"Get out here, coward!" Robert screamed.

No response. Robert wheeled. Joaquin came fast at him, three yards away. Robert threw himself forward like a catapulted boulder and head-butted Joaquin's orbital bone, turning his head sideways. The move gave Robert time to rear back once more and head-butt the man's temporal bone.

Down the mass-murderer went, his already-jittery brain shorting out.

Exhausted, Robert melted to the floor. Joaquin stared at him, his head twitching, his eyes trembling. Robert slid his legs around Joaquin's throat and started to squeeze with all the might he had left, snapping Joaquin's cervical vertebrae into pieces.

"You killed Joaquin!" came a voice from behind him. "You're going to pay, *hijo de puta!*"

Robert turned. Pablo was ten yards away, pressing his heavy boot down on Guillermo's neck. He was a middle-aged man but no bigger than a grade-schooler, sporting a pathetic wispy mustache. He held Robert's heavy Sig with a rock-steady hand. He pointed the gun at Guillermo's temple and prepared to pull the trigger.

"No! Please don't!" Robert screamed. "It's over, man. We'll let you escape. I promise, we won't go after you."

Pablo merely gazed down casually. "Now that Joaquin is gone, I get to take over."

"Let him go."

"And after I get rid of you guys, I won't have to look over my shoulder."

"No!" Robert yelled again, as Pablo leaned forward and pulled the trigger.

Robert shut his eyes and braced for what he knew would be worse than losing his own life.

CHAPTER 50

A familiar wheeze made Robert's eyes spring open.

A carbon-dark arrow pierced Pablo's chest. He fell back and shot the gun into the half-collapsed ceiling.

Then he clutched the arrow as blood pulsed from the wound.

Guillermo's hand snaked around Pablo's stumbling foot, heaving it from under him. Pablo froze as whatever animated him left.

And there was Mel, holding Robert's prized bow and arrows. He walked toward Robert and peered at him like a concerned doctor. "You okay?"

"I am now. It's great to see you, amigo."

Mel rushed over to the medical cabinet, grabbed some bandages, and ran back to Robert.

"Jesus," Mel cried, as he wrapped Robert's wounded leg. "How are you even standing?"

Robert tried to smile, but a geyser of total fatigue shot up his spine. It whooshed away his sense of balance and plopped him on his butt. "Help Guillermo." He pointed at Joaquin. "Handcuffs. Keys. Back pocket."

Mel rifled through the dead man's pockets until he found a small ring of keys. In minutes all cuffs were off.

"Welcome to the dark side," Guillermo rasped, grinning. "Your first kill was a good one."

"I'm just glad I got here in time." Mel moved closer to Guillermo's face, squinting into his eyes. "You got some periorbital edema and ecchymosis over that lac." He handed Guillermo a packet of sterile gauze.

Guillermo took it and placed a bunch over the open wound. "I had a brief go-round with a garbage disposal."

Doc trotted inside the warehouse. When he reached Robert's side, he sat back on his haunches, panting. His fur was covered with dust and microdebris from the explosion.

Robert reached down and stroked the dog's back, delighted to see him.

Guillermo stood. "I need a vacation."

Robert regained some of his lost energy. "How did you find us, Mel?"

"I was in the lobby of the hotel waiting for a cab to take me to the airport, so I decided to call New York. As soon as I got off the phone with Rivera, I ran to your room, hoping to catch you guys before you left on your mission. I saw the map on your bed and the bow and arrow set. I didn't have a gun, so I figured I'd come in armed."

"What did Rivera say that made you so concerned?" Guillermo asked.

"Is it Francine?" Robert asked.

"No, no, not at all," Mel stammered. "She's actually recovering, Robert. Following commands. Answering questions appropriately." He sighed. "You were right. She admitted to overdosing on Ambien."

Robert nodded but didn't say anything.

"Then what?" Guillermo asked.

"Rivera couldn't get into it," Mel explained. "All she said was that someone called the ER yesterday asking for you,

Robert. It sounded urgent. They instructed her to get in touch with you as soon as possible, told her to make sure you checked your e-mail." Mel looked into Robert's eyes. "She said the guy told her it was a matter of life and death."

"My e-mail?" Robert repeated.

"Who would want to get in touch with you so badly?" Guillermo asked.

"Maybe a family member?" Mel suggested.

Robert gazed blankly at Mel. "I have no living relatives."

"No sense in wasting time speculating," Guillermo said. "Let's get your stuff out of the bank deposit box and find out."

CHAPTER 51

Robert collected his computer and cellphone from where he'd left them in the Guatemala City Bank safe deposit box. He started to open the laptop in the vault, but hesitated. Better to be with Guillermo. Rivera wasn't the type to be dramatic. If she said this was an emergency, Robert didn't doubt it.

He headed across the street to the café where Guillermo, Mel, and Doc waited. The cellphone seemed to writhe in his pocket like a dying rat; the laptop under his arm felt like a pressure bomb he had to keep from going off by squeezing it tighter and tighter.

"Calm your mind," Guillermo told him the moment he arrived. "No need to breathe less."

The sound of his mentor's words immediately relaxed Robert, and he took a cleansing breath. "Let's move away from everyone, away from the windows."

As they maneuvered through the crowd at the bar, Mel said to Robert, "Plane leaves in two hours. We've got a car coming for us."

They sat at a table in an unlit row in the back, Doc curled beneath.

Robert fired up his laptop.

Clicked on e-mail.

They all stared as Robert scrolled through weeks of useless spam and a few notes from acquaintances. Finally he came to a dozen from the same address.

Same subject.

The Owl's Revenge.

Sent every hour on the hour starting the night before last.

Robert fingered the pointer to a link on the most recent e-mail.

He tapped the touchpad twice.

A video.

At first there was nothing but darkness. Then the darkness throbbed to different shades of black that morphed into red.

An eye.

The camera backed up. The red eye belonged to a large, dark-brown feathered owl. The camera followed this eye as the head turned completely around, then blinked with malevolent slowness.

The owl flew away, its wings spreading beautifully across a moonlit sky. Robert heard the sound of hooting, growing faint.

Then a blare.

And his nightmare began.

Robert saw Sharon with her hands and feet roped to the four corners of a bed, loosely clad in lingerie.

Her face and arms bruised.

And the insides of her thighs.

Her mouth was duct-taped, her eyes wide with her struggle to get enough air.

A dark figure in a hooded black robe and black gloves, wearing large glasses to emulate the eyes of an owl, came before the camera and hooted three times with a smile on his face. He walked over to Sharon and stroked his gloved fingers up the inside of her thighs, cupped her crotch and squeezed tightly, then slowly moved his hand to her abdomen and breasts. He stroked her cheek. As he did Sharon's gaze seemed to project from her eyes thousands of miles per second into Robert's and he saw a fierceness, a diamond resolve to last long enough for Robert to help her dismember this creep.

With a display of force, the man pulled back and backhanded Sharon, knocking her unconscious.

Robert fought to calm his pounding heart.

The man stuck his head close to the camera, showing only his large sunglasses and fake owl-beak nose. His voice was distorted mechanically, a favorite kidnapper's device, so that he sounded like a bullhorn with a dying battery.

"You're probably wondering who I am?" A feminine, sinister laugh. "Who am I, Dr. McKenzie? A clue. I'm in your memory, and now I'm setting up my nest there. I'm all the horrible things you've done that you don't want to remember. I'm all the evil from your past rolled into someone who wants you to feel all the horror you've made others feel. You ruined all the joy I ever found, everything I devoted my life to. You shoved me into a maze where nothing was friendly, and my constant, growing dread was nothing compared to the dreadful realities attacking me at every turn. You're going to get a lesson in compassion. Your precious Sharon"—the Owl turned back and stared at Sharon's unconscious form spread-eagled on the four-poster—"will be raped over and over, and tormented to death with infinite slowness. All on camera. For everyone in the world to see. The most viral video ever. And we will find closure, you and I. You will finally experience the healthy catharsis of fully embracing your dark side, and I will finally purge myself of an obsession that will not leave me until I get my revenge."

He stared into the video camera.

"My obsession is to avenge what you once did to me, Dr. McKenzie. Today you get to crack the mystery of time and learn the deepest secrets so long hidden in the darkness of your heart."

A picture of a calendar and a date circled in red ink.

It was three days away.

"If you don't find me by Sunday at midnight, lovely Sharon will begin to lose her loveliness—and her mind. She will beg for her life by the time the Owl is through with her. Get here in time and she'll survive—crippled, no doubt, for the rest of her life, but alive. Are we clear, Dr. McKenzie? Or should I say, Dr. Vigilante?"

Then the video went dead.

Robert started hyperventilating. An electric whine sawed through his brain.

"Robert!" Guillermo shook him by the shoulders, bringing his eyes back in focus. "Look at me. Deep breaths. Deep, slow breaths."

The sound of Guillermo's voice drowned out the buzzing.

"Sharon needs you to focus," Guillermo instructed. "Deep breaths. Reach her with your breaths. Think of her looking to you, trusting you. Breathe that. Breathe Sharon. Breathe in: *Sharon.* Breathe out: *I'm coming.* That's it."

"I'm coming."

"That's it."

Robert nodded, breathing deeply again. He closed his eyes but the obscenity of Sharon on the bed immediately came up, and he had to jolt his eyes back open. The image faded. He forced himself to breathe slower and longer. As he did, he imagined her eyes reaching out to his, and he willed the image to stay strong.

He felt his sanity floating back down from the spinning sky. Though his mind still raced, he could pull from its deafening babel the questions he needed to answer.

Do I know this guy? Was he one of the neo-Nazis I put down? Or a relative of one of the many wife-abusers I've maimed?

Why does he call me Dr. Vigilante? What does he know about me? How do I find him?

Is Sharon already beyond help?

All these thoughts rat-a-tatted through his mind in seconds. He took another breath and turned down the volume inside. Three breaths later, he found a workable quiet.

One thing at a time, one step after the other.

"I'm going to find this guy," he said.

"No doubt," Mel said. "But how?"

"He wants me to. He'll leave clues because he's smug and stupid."

"Scavenger hunt," Guillermo said.

"Right," Robert said. "And I'm going to scavenge the hell out of that motherfucker."

"I can't come with you," Guillermo said. "But you don't want me to."

"You have plenty to do," Robert said. "You have to put your people back together again."

"Car's here," Mel said.

Robert stood.

Guillermo hugged him. "Stay focused."

"I will."

"What are you going to do?" Guillermo asked.

"Find the Owl."

"And when you do?"

Robert gritted his teeth. "And when I do, God help him."

Made in the USA
Monee, IL
04 November 2026

67377202R00164